7-11-02

Compliments of
Boehringer Ingelheim
pharmaceuticals, Inc
- Jeff ~~Martin~~
~~817 933 4370~~, 8722#
Aggrenox
Mirapex

D0119251

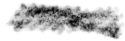

An Atlas of
STROKE
2nd edition

THE ENCYCLOPEDIA OF VISUAL MEDICINE SERIES

An Atlas of
STROKE
2nd edition

Peter F. Semple, MB, FRCP

Senior Lecturer and Consultant Physician
Department of Medicine & Therapeutics, Gardiner Institute
Western Infirmary, Glasgow, Scotland, UK

and

Ralph L. Sacco, MS, MD

Associate Professor of Neurology and Public Health
Associate Chairman of Neurology, Columbia University
College of Physicians and Surgeons, New York, NY, USA

Foreword by

Justin A. Zivin, MD, PhD

Professor of Neurosciences, School of Medicine
University of California, San Diego
La Jolla, CA, USA

The Parthenon Publishing Group
International Publishers in Medicine, Science & Technology

NEW YORK   LONDON

Library of Congress Cataloging-in-Publication Data

Semple, Peter F.

    An atlas of stroke / Peter F. Semple and Ralph L. Sacco :
foreword by Justin A. Zivin. -- 2nd ed.

       p. cm. -- (The encyclopedia of visual medicine series)
    Includes bibliographical references and index.
    ISBN 1-85070-082-6
    1. Cerebrovascular disease Atlases. I. Sacco, Ralph L. II.
Title. III. Series.
    [DNLM: 1. Cerebrovascular Disorders atlases. WL 17
S473a 1999]
RC388.5.S455 1999
616.8'1--dc21
DNLM/DLC
for Library of Congress   99–14700
                                    CIP

British Library Cataloguing in Publication Data

Semple, Peter F.

    An atlas of stroke. - 2nd ed. - (The encyclopedia of visual
medicine series)
    1. Cerebrovascular disease 2. Cerebrovascular disease -
Diagnosis 3. Cerebrovascular disease - Treatment
    I. Title II. Sacco, Ralph L.
    616.8'1

    ISBN 1-85070-082-6

Published in the USA by
The Parthenon Publishing Group Inc.
One Blue Hill Plaza
PO Box 1564, Pearl River
New York 10965, USA

Published in the UK and Europe by
The Parthenon Publishing Group Limited
Casterton Hall, Carnforth
Lancs. LA6 2LA, UK

Copyright ©1999 Parthenon Publishing Group

Printed and bound in Spain by T.G. Hostench, S.A.

Contents

Foreword

Until about a quarter of a century ago, all that we physicians could do for the cerebrovascular patient was to classify the various types of strokes. The actual treatment of stroke was an unattainable dream. Diagnosis was occasionally extremely challenging, and localization was based on clinical rules that sometimes failed.

The first revolution in the management of patients with cerebrovascular disease came when imaging methods were markedly improved. There are now a number of techniques that are helpful, and even more sophisticated modalities can be anticipated in the future. Diagnosis is now rarely difficult to achieve and stroke localization is precise.

Around two decades ago, stroke therapy began to be truly effective. Until that time, many therapeutic decisions were based on anecdotal evidence and 'armchair speculation' of a type that has now been shown to be useless or even worse. More recently, laboratory investigations and well-conducted clinical trials have provided a scientific basis for stroke treatment. First to come from this knowledge were the various prophylactic therapies. Hypertension control was shown to be important.

This was followed by proof that antiplatelet therapy is useful. Subsequently, the roles of surgical therapies and anticoagulation have become more clearly defined. The most recent steps forward have been towards the development of effective acute stroke therapies.

Strokes are one of the most common causes of death and disability in many parts of the world, and there is increasing emphasis on the need for speed in initiation of therapy. Therefore, many types of physicians will need to become familiar and comfortable with dealing with this disease. With this atlas, the authors have written a simple but up-to-date summary of the rapidly advancing field of clinical imaging technology for the diagnosis and management of stroke patients. This book should provide students and physicians who are not cerebrovascular specialists with a sound foundation for an understanding of modern diagnostic procedures and the current literature. The concept of stroke therapy is no longer an oxymoron, and dissemination of the information contained in this atlas should be helpful to those of us who care for such patients.

Justin A. Zivin
La Jolla

Acknowledgements

I am grateful to the following colleagues for generously allowing the use of their slides in this atlas:

Dr Fred Adams, Dr Michael Sproule, Dr Tom Barrie, Dr John Byrne, Professor Henry Dargie and Mr Ian Sim of the Western Infirmary, Glasgow, Scotland;

Dr Marie Callaghan of the Law Hospital, Carluke, Lanarkshire; and

Dr Donald Grossett and Dr Keith Muir of the Institute of Neurological Sciences, Southern General Hospital, Glasgow, Scotland.

I would also like to thank Dr Alan S. Cohen of the Boston University School of Medicine, Boston, Massachusetts, USA, who so kindly provided the histological slides of amyloid angiopathy.

Finally, I am grateful to my colleagues, medical illustrators and all the others who have helped to make the idea of this present volume a reality.

Peter F. Semple
Glasgow

I wish to thank Alexander G. Khandji, MD, Vice Chairman and Associate Director of Radiology, Associate Professor of Radiology, College of Physicians and Surgeons of Columbia University, New York, for providing the magnetic resonance imaging scans used in Figures 17, 19, 23, 24 and 35.

Ralph L. Sacco
New York

Preface

At the time I was training as a physician in the early seventies, the diagnosis of stroke was solely clinical, supplemented on occasions by lumbar punctures and angiography, both of which were often embarked upon with trepidation.

The advent of computed tomography in the early seventies changed everything, not least because the technology permitted rapid, accurate and immediate diagnosis of hemorrhage. In the eighties came magnetic resonance imaging, which has greatly extended the ability to diagnose ischemic stroke, and produces remarkable images of the living brain. At the same time, Doppler ultrasound has evolved into an indispensable technique for the diagnosis of carotid artery disease. Other non-invasive methods of imaging the vasculature of the brain are being improved by the day.

The routine care of the acute stroke patient has improved greatly since my early years as a practicing physician. Moreover, I believe that we are now on the threshold of an exciting new era when effective treatment will at last be possible, probably in the form of early thrombolysis and novel neuroprotective drugs. Such an era will be in sharp contrast to the atmosphere of nihilism that appeared to prevail during earlier years.

The prevention of stroke by the use of antihypertensive and antithrombotic agents is now firmly established, and supported by incontrovertible evidence of efficacy. The main challenge remaining is to ensure that appropriate and effective pharmaceutical treatment is delivered to those at particular risk due to high blood pressure and atrial fibrillation, among other medical conditions.

The images of stroke now available from modern investigative technologies are striking and lend themselves particularly well to visual display in an atlas. *An Atlas of Stroke* is a logical extension from my earlier book, *An Atlas of Hypertension*.

I hope that this present atlas, as with its earlier 'partner', will prove to be a useful aid to those clinicians who are involved in the management of patients with vascular disorders.

Peter F. Semple
Glasgow

Section 1 A Review of Stroke

Epidemiology

Louis Pasteur sustained a left hemiparesis due to stroke at the age of 43 years. Fortunately, his intellect was apparently not impaired as he continued his celebrated research on microorganisms which culminated in the famous description of immunization against rabies.

Stroke, or apoplexy as it was once known, is the third leading cause of death in the developed world. It is, however, perhaps better known as a major cause of disability, accounting for no less than 5% of all monetary expenditure on health.

The condition is usually relatively easy to recognize clinically, as reflected by the definition of the World Health Organization (WHO): '...rapidly developing clinical signs of focal (or global) disturbance of cerebral function with symptoms lasting 24 hours or longer or leading to death with no apparent cause other than of vascular origin.' This definition encompasses subarachnoid hemorrhage, a distinctive condition with a unique pathophysiology and treatment.

Based on surveys of incidence and survival, the prevalence of stroke in the general population is 500–700 / 100 000 population, of whom at least half are left physically disabled or intellectually impaired[1]. The incidence increases exponentially with age from around 200 / 100 000 in the decade spanning the age of 60 years to around 3000 / 100 000 after age 85 years. There is some variation from country to country so that, after age 65 years, almost 90% of deaths are caused by stroke[2,3].

In most developed countries, the rate of mortality has fallen progressively over the century, with Japan showing a particularly steep decline. The annual rate of fall in the United States has tended to be around 5% in recent years, which appears to be due more to a reduction in case–fatality rate rather than in incidence. Small cohort studies suggest that the incidence fell in eastern parts of the USA between the late 1940s and 1970s, and a similar decline was observed in Japan over the decade spanning the 1960s. In contrast, there is evidence from Eastern Europe to suggest that the incidence in those aged <70 years may in fact be increasing, despite the expected reduction in case–fatality rate[4].

Apparent increases in incidence in the USA more recently[5] must be viewed with some skepticism as diagnosis has improved with the advent of computed tomography (CT), and with the advances in this and other imaging techniques. Secular trends are always subject to potential bias due to changes in clinical practice and more subtle changes in diagnostic criteria. Furthermore, any changes in incidence and case–fatality rate must be viewed in the light of demographic changes resulting from increases in life expectancy and differing race–ethnic distributions.

The American Heart Association and the US National Stroke Association have estimated that there are nearly 4 000 000 survivors of stroke in the USA and around 155 000 deaths due to stroke each year[6,7]. Recent updated projections have estimated that nearly 700 000 strokes occur each year. By the year 2050, more than 1 000 000 Americans per year may experience a stroke.

The WHO-sponsored MONICA project has established stroke registration in representative groups of the populations of 15 countries since 1984. The information is linked to the collection of data on risk factors and other cardiovascular events, and should provide a better idea of the more recent trends in incidence. In general and across different countries, it appears that stroke mortality tends to be higher where coronary heart disease mortality is lower.

The burden on the community is heavy. In particular, the costs of managing acute stroke are likely to increase now that there is good evidence to suggest that acute stroke units linked to a wider range of imaging techniques can reduce case–fatality rates. Around one-fifth of the patients who survive stroke require institutional care for the remainder of their lives. Stroke is also the terminal event for many elderly patients who are already disabled or in care so that up to 40% of stroke patients die in hospital.

Classification

Stroke may be classified into three distinct groups: subarachnoid hemorrhage; intracerebral hemorrhage; and cerebral infarction. Subarachnoid hemorrhage has a characteristic presentation, affects younger patients and accounts for around 5% of strokes. Intracerebral hemorrhage is easily detected on CT, but is a relatively infrequent cause of stroke; at present, bleeding accounts for around 10–15% of admissions to an acute stroke unit both in Europe and in North America. The pattern in the Far East is somewhat different, with intracerebral hemorrhage accounting for around 25% of strokes in Japan. Such differences are probably the result of different patterns of risk factors in the respective populations, particularly arterial blood pressure, and plasma levels of cholesterol and other lipid fractions.

A reliable subclassification of cerebral infarction is more difficult to determine because various processes lead to interruption of blood flow, including atherosclerosis and thrombosis, small-vessel disease and embolism, which itself can be further divided into cardiac embolism and artery-to-artery embolism.

Various schemes for a clinical classification of stroke have been devised, supplemented or confirmed by information from CT, magnetic resonance imaging (MRI), carotid duplex Doppler ultrasonography or other imaging techniques.

The Oxford scheme of clinical classification (see Section 2, Figure 1) is widely used[8], and divides infarcts into carotid or anterior circulation infarcts (ACI) and vertebrobasilar or posterior circulation infarcts (POCI). The ACI are further subdivided into lesions which affect both cortical and subcortical structures, resulting in hemiplegia, hemisensory loss, hemianopia and higher cortical dysfunction, and are referred to as total ACI or TACI. Events which cause only partial cortical deficits, such as aphasia, are referred to as partial ACI or PACI.

The Oxford classification is useful in terms of prognosis as total syndromes have a poor prognosis for survival and functional outcome. However, the scheme does not distinguish between embolic and atherothrombotic events.

Since the pioneering studies of C. Miller Fisher in Boston, lacunar infarcts (or LACI in the Oxford system) have been delineated by clinical criteria based on neuroanatomical principles[9]. Lacunar infarcts were originally defined as events resulting from occlusion of single perforating end arteries 50–200 Å in diameter. The definition remains useful in clinical practice in terms of prognosis and definition of subgroups for clinical trials. Its main weakness is the incomplete relationship to pathophysiology as small deep infarcts may also be a result of atherosclerosis as well as of the characteristic small-vessel disease of hypertension and diabetes mellitus. Some posterior circulation infarcts are lacunar and share a common patho-physiology.

Other classification schemes have been devised and are based more on pathological, rather than neuroanatomical, mechanisms. These include that derived from data from the Stroke Data Bank Study[10] and that of the National Institute of Neurological Disorders and Stroke[11] (see Section 2, Figures 1 and 2). Both systems infer causality on the basis of the presence of potential cardiac sources of embolism and of proximal arterial stenoses. In clinical practice, however, such a distinction is not easily achieved and there is often no entirely reliable method of verification. Some of the common and less common causes of acute ischemic stroke and transient ischemic attacks (TIAs) are shown in Section 2, Figure 3.

Neuronal ischemia and the ischemic penumbra

Deficient blood supply to a part of the brain causes reduced function of neurons and glia which may progress to cell death and permanent dysfunction. The biochemical mechanisms of ischemia and cell death have been extensively investigated, focusing on strategies and treatments that may prevent or attenuate permanent damage. Brain ischemia affects not only neurotransmitters, receptors, membrane ion channels and processes of phosphorylation, but may also have an effect on the generation of toxic free radicals as well as on modification of gene expression and regulation. Neurons and glial cells are affected in different ways, and there is particular interest in processes that may be reversible.

Certain neurons, namely, the pyramidal neurons in the CA1 and CA4 zones of the hippocampus, and some of the neurons in the caudate nucleus, are most vulnerable to ischemic death. Histopathology after cardiac arrest in animals has provided information regarding the vulnerability of neurons to global ischemia, and focal ischemia could be expected to have similar effects. A period of 60 min or less of focal ischemia is sufficient to cause infarction and necrosis of neurons and glia, but there is a surrounding zone of spared glia. Around the central area of necrosis is an area of ischemia causing cell dysfunction of variable degrees, some of which are potentially reversible. Severe ischemia causes persistent depolarization of neurons, but there is a surrounding zone of only intermittent depolarization. This area is often described as the ischemic penumbra and may vary considerably in size.

Severe ischemia causes depletion of adenosine triphosphate (ATP), but energy failure is probably not the immediate cause of cell necrosis. Other downstream factors may kill cells either immediately or after a period of time, even when the initial ATP levels have been restored. Generation of toxic free radical species as a result of ischemia and reperfusion may be a critical mechanism determining cell injury and death, but acidosis due in part to lactate accumulation is also a mediator of cell injury, particularly in the neuroglia.

Failure of energy supplies to the ion pumps that maintain membrane potential levels results in a collapse of gradients of sodium, potassium and calcium across cells, and an increase in intracellular calcium, with resultant calcium mediator-enzyme activation; this has also been implicated as a cause of cell death. Thus far, however, it has been disappointing that attempts to prevent cell death by blockade of calcium entry or intracellular release of calcium have not been entirely successful.

Intracellular and excitatory amino acids such as glutamate, glycine and aspartate are released in response to ischemia. Various studies have provided evidence that calcium entry through glutamate-regulated membrane channels is detrimental to survival. Several receptors appear to be involved, including the quisqualate and NMDA (*N*-methyl-D-aspartate) receptor complexes which are linked to calcium entry channels.

In animal models of acute ischemic stroke, ultimate infarct size can be substantially attenuated by the administration of several experimental agents either before or after arterial occlusion. In addition, as in the heart, there appears to be an ischemic tolerance phenomenon[12]. Tolerance of ischemia in the brain apparently develops more slowly and persists for longer than in the heart, and probably requires the synthesis of new protein.

A major challenge for clinical trials is to administer potentially effective agents as early as possible after the onset of ischemia and to deliver the drug in adequate concentrations to the tissue that has a reduced blood supply. For clinical trials of neuroprotective drugs, the inhomogeneous nature of acute stroke in humans creates further difficulties. Ischemic stroke may be the result of large-artery thrombosis, small-vessel disease affecting subcortical white matter, embolism from the heart or proximal arteries and various other rare vascular events, including arterial dissection and arteritis.

Transient ischemic attacks (TIAs)

The time-honored definition of a TIA is an episode of focal loss of cerebral function or vision lasting <24 h due to a temporary interruption of blood supply. A TIA is a precursor of stroke as around one in three patients who present with TIA will develop completed stroke within 3 years. The clinical syndrome identifies a group of patients in some of whom stroke may be prevented by treatment of a carotid stenosis or by institution of antithrombotic measures or, less frequently, by diagnosis of conditions such as systemic lupus erythematosus or necrotizing arteritis.

Symptoms of cerebral dysfunction that are not focal, such as confusion, loss of consciousness or loss of vision associated with a reduced level of consciousness, are not considered TIAs. Likewise, isolated symptoms that may have other causes, such as vertigo and disturbances of balance, dysarthria and dysphagia, scintillating scotomas and sensory symptoms confined to part of a limb or the face, are also not classified under the rubric.

Migraine and seizures are often considered in the differential diagnosis, although migraine with aura may present particular difficulties. In migraine, there tends to be a slow progression of symptoms from part to part over a period of up to 30 min, and affected patients tend to be relatively young. Headache is not a particularly useful discriminant.

In contrast, focal seizures tend to cause 'positive' rather than 'negative' symptoms, and have a characteristic rapid progression from a distal point in the limb or face to become more widespread.

A TIA due to a critical carotid stenosis may occasionally cause shaking or tremor of a limb which may be mistaken for a focal seizure. TIAs in the carotid territory tend to cause visual loss in one eye, aphasia or unilateral motor and / or sensory symptoms. However, some posterior circulation events may have similar presentations.

Sensory or motor symptoms that are bilateral suggest that ischemia in the vertebrobasilar territory is highly likely as do blindness, diplopia, vertigo and loss of balance.

Patient history and clinical examination may give useful pointers as to the mechanism of TIAs. Bruits may be detected over the carotid artery and, less commonly, the subclavian artery, but tend not to be either sensitive or specific. Systolic murmurs transmitted from the aortic valve may lead to false-positive results.

The familiar description of symptoms of hemispheric ischemia or amaurosis fugax should prompt carotid Doppler ultrasonography to establish the presence of carotid atherosclerosis and stenosis. In such cases, CT and MRI are of limited value for investigation as it is often difficult to date stroke events with certainty, and brain-stem infarcts are difficult to visualize with CT. Although these imaging modalities are a necessary component of patient investigation, most clinicians continue to define the condition solely on the basis of clinical criteria.

Atrial fibrillation, cardiac murmurs or evidence of myocardial infarction should raise suspicions of cardiogenic embolism, and electrocardiography (ECG) and echocardiography may provide similar clues.

Transthoracic echocardiography is especially effective in identifying left ventricular dysfunction and ventricular sources of embolism, but has limited value in detecting thrombus in the atria and atrial appendages, for which the transesophageal echocardiography (TEE) approach provides much better definition. TEE is also able to render good definition of the aorta and may give a diagnosis of dissection or reveal evidence of a protruding atheroma, a potential source of atheroembolism.

Artery-to-artery embolism may give rise to refractile deposits in the retinal arterioles, so-called Hollenhorst plaques, which tend to be visualized at points of arteriolar bifurcation. Finally, uncontrolled hypertension may be a pointer to an incipient lacunar event.

Brain imaging using CT or MRI may reveal evidence of previous events. MRI is better than CT in detecting brain-stem infarction and small deep hemispheric infarcts. Cerebrovascular ischemic changes can be detected earlier with MRI, although small bright signals may be present and give false-positive results. The requirement for the patient to remain still and recumbent in an MRI scanner is a major limitation on acute use, and claustrophobia may sometimes cause difficulties.

Large-artery atherosclerosis

The presence of infarcts between areas supplied by different cerebral arteries may be an indication of a period of reduced cerebral perfusion or suggest the presence of a proximal arterial stenosis. The most easily recognizable border-zone or 'watershed' infarcts are located between the territories of the middle and anterior, and middle and posterior, cerebral arteries, although variability in blood supply from one individual to another can lead to difficulties in recognition. Infarcts at the junctions of deep and superficial middle cerebral arterial branches, and in the cerebellar hemisphere, are more difficult to recognize.

Ultrasound is widely used as a screening test for carotid atherosclerosis and stenosis, and is particularly appropriate in the investigation of ischemic symptoms of the anterior cerebral circulation and eye[13,14]. Nowadays, carotid revascularization may not require prior contrast arteriography[15] and non-invasive approaches such as MRI angiography and spiral CT may be useful in defining arterial anatomy.

Over the last 20 years, there has been a major increase in the technology of carotid ultrasonography. Advances have included increased selectivity and sensitivity of pulsed Doppler ultrasound, the addition of color imaging and improved resolution.

Duplex sonography describes the combination of ultrasound imaging of the vessel wall with pulse-gated Doppler. The procedures are linked so that the two-dimensional real-time image can be used to locate the area of interest for the Doppler part of the study. The duplex system allows the operator to switch easily from one mode to the other. Doppler signatures are digitized and visually displayed.

Occlusion of the internal carotid artery can now be diagnosed with added confidence by Doppler with color-coded flow velocities (CDI). Additional information regarding plaque morphology, and especially ulceration and hemorrhage, can be obtained with an acceptable degree of accuracy. The technique has also been used to quantify intima–media thickness (IMT) as an index of atherosclerosis in clinical trials. However, a major limitation of all ultrasound systems is the inability to detect 'tandem' lesions in the carotid siphon or middle cerebral artery. Transcranial Doppler and MRI angiography may be useful non-invasive methods for detecting middle cerebral artery stenosis. With Doppler, there is a small risk (1–10%) that high-grade internal carotid stenoses may be mistaken for total occlusion and, thus, many prefer to make a precise assessment of arterial anatomy with contrast angiography. Another non-invasive screening technique for internal carotid stenosis is ocular pneumoplethysmography, although the method has not found much favor.

The mechanism of cerebral ischemia in carotid stenosis is thought to involve artery-to-artery embolism in the majority of cases, although ischemic events secondary to hemodynamic changes are seen. The latter tend to be stereotyped and are liable to be provoked by reductions in arterial pressure or cardiac output.

The major clinical studies of carotid endarterectomy for symptomatic internal carotid stenosis that have guided current clinical practice are the European Carotid Stenosis Trial (ECST), the Veterans Administration Symptomatic Trial and the North American Symptomatic Carotid Endarterectomy Trial (NASCET) published in 1991[16-18]. More recently, the Asymptomatic Carotid Atherosclerosis Study (ACAS) on the surgical management of asymptomatic stenosis has reported positive results[19].

There are a number of methodological problems because of the different systems used to quantify the degree of arterial stenosis in the different trials. All of the various methods used calculated the percentage of minimal residual lumen (MRL), but different denominators were applied, such as the distal lumen (DL) diameter or 'normal' bulb diameter. Further uncertainty has resulted from the use of various definitions for the carotid bulb and sinus, and it has also been suggested that the diameter of the proximal common carotid artery may be a better reference point.

In practice, most clinicians use the diameter of the MRL divided by the diameter of the DL, where the walls are parallel. However, diameter stenosis in one plane is not linearly related to a cross-sectional area. Therefore, a 50% diameter stenosis approximates to a 75% area stenosis. The relationship between angiographic and Doppler measurements in a given laboratory is not always well-defined and may be another potential pitfall in the assessment of severity.

Distal stenosis and restenosis after surgery may be treated by angioplasty and stent, but the roles of these newer techniques are currently still not fully defined. A prospective randomized clinical trial comparing surgery with angioplasty and stent insertion is necessary before the uses of these less invasive techniques can be assessed. Uncontrolled use of catheter-based methods may not be appropriate at present.

Earlier hopes that intravenous digital subtraction angiography might replace intra-arterial contrast injection have not been realized because the quality of the former image tends to be less than optimal, especially if left ventricular function is impaired. MRI angiography and spiral CT are promising, but large-scale experience has not yet been accumulated and image definition remains inferior to that achieved with intra-arterial contrast injection.

There is a general consensus that surgical treatment can provide benefit in suitable patients who have severe symptomatic stenosis (>70%), but there is much less agreement regarding the cost-effectiveness of treating asymptomatic patients. For a single ischemic event and compared with medical treatment, surgery reduces the risk of ipsilateral stroke at 2 years from 19% to 9%, and that of recurrent events from 41% to 11%[20]. It is recognized that surgeons who carry out endarterectomy need to perform sufficient numbers of procedures to verify the rate of complications in terms of operative morbidity; stroke morbidity should be around 2% and certainly less than 5%.

The most important approach to the medical management of carotid stenosis is the use of antiplatelet drugs. In the most recent meta-analysis of stroke risk reduction in patients with TIAs or minor ischemic stroke, antiplatelet drugs resulted in a 2% absolute-risk reduction and a 23% odds reduction in terms of non-fatal stroke[21]. Furthermore, both the new antiplatelet drug clopidogrel and the combination of extended-release dipyridamole plus aspirin may be more effective than aspirin alone[22,23]. The optimal dose of aspirin for stroke prophylaxis remains the subject of intense debate[24,25]; however, the US Food and Drug Administration has recommended doses of 50–325 mg of aspirin for persons with stroke or TIA.

Other experimental techniques may provide useful information regarding cerebral perfusion distal to an extracranial or intracranial arterial stenosis. Changes in flow velocity within the middle cerebral artery, as determined by transcranial Doppler ultrasound, may allow assessment of hemispheric perfusion reserve. The reserve will be reduced if flow velocity remains unaffected by elevation of arterial carbon dioxide partial pressure (pCO_2), which is accomplished simply by breath-holding.

Another technique for quantifying hemispheric blood flow is single-photon emission computed tomography (SPECT), which uses the gamma-emitting properties of radioligands such as technetium 99m (^{99m}Tc)-hexamethylpropylene amine oxide (HMPAO) or [123]I (radioiodine)-amphetamine, and produces images using a standard gamma camera. Scanning during ischemia may provide information concerning distribution. Investigation can be carried out before and after manipulation of pCO_2 by acetazolamide treatment to allow estimation of perfusion reserve. The advent of perfusion MRI may also be an adjunct to the evaluation of large-artery atherosclerosis in patients with cerebral ischemia. However, these techniques are not as yet used routinely in the investigation of TIAs and stroke.

Cardioembolism

Embolism from the heart as a cause of stroke was first recognized nearly 150 years ago. The entity has attracted increasing attention during the last decade because of several clinical trials which have clearly demonstrated the benefit of anticoagulant treatment in preventing stroke in patients with potential cardiac sources, especially atrial fibrillation.

At present, there is no certain method for differentiating embolic stroke from other types of arterial occlusion. It has been estimated that embolism accounts for 15–20% of clinical stroke events[26,27]. Mode of onset is sometimes helpful in that slow or stuttering onset is clearly not consistent with an embolic etiology. Major risk factors include atrial fibrillation, anterior myocardial infarction, a poorly contracting left ventricle[28] and mitral valve disease.

The advent of TEE has given impetus to the search for potential sources in the heart. In series of patients with acute stroke, potential embolic sources have been recognized in up to one-third of patients[29]. Unfortunately, patients with a risk of embolism due to atrial fibrillation often have concomitant ischemic or hypertensive heart disease and cranial or extracranial atherosclerosis.

Embolism tends to be more frequently a cause of stroke in the very young, who should be subjected to careful cardiac investigation. However, embolism is also relatively frequent in elderly patients with stroke, a group in whom the recognition of embolism is much more difficult and where the risks of anticoagulant treatment must be carefully weighed against the known benefits.

The type and location of infarction, as seen on CT, is sometimes helpful in diagnosis. Embolism from the atria or ventricles tends to cause cortical infarcts, including some of the middle cerebral artery branch syndromes, especially occlusion at the first branch of the lower division, resulting in Wernicke's aphasia, as well as posterior cerebral artery occlusion. Striatocapsular infarcts are also likely to have an embolic cause as sudden occlusion of the cerebral artery stem will block the orifices of the lenticulostriate arteries with relative sparing of superficial middle cerebral artery territories.

Smaller subcortical events of lacunar type are not currently believed to result from embolism. The distribution of injected microspheres in experimental animals offers some support to this view.

Early hemorrhagic transformation of cerebral infarcts is somewhat more likely after embolic stroke, although reperfusion and hemorrhage may also develop in large infarcts caused by atherosclerosis. Indeed, nearly 40% of middle cerebral artery infarcts show some evidence of reperfusion at 48 h.

Multiple cortical infarcts in an elderly patient in the presence of a cardiac source strongly suggest an embolic cause whereas embolism from heart valves tends to cause TIAs or amaurosis fugax. In patients with mechanical prosthetic heart valves, prophylaxis may be best if warfarin is combined with low-dose aspirin. The benefits of such a combination appear to outweigh the increased risk of gastro-intestinal bleeding[30], although some argue that optimal control of anticoagulation with warfarin alone achieves the same results.

The risk of embolism in young patients is probably increased in the presence of mitral valve prolapse, patent foramen ovale and atrial septal aneurysm[31]. Transcranial Doppler sonography after intravenous injection of microbubbles, perhaps supplemented by cough or the Valsalva maneuver, is useful for detecting those who have patent foramen ovale or, alternatively, TEE[32].

Other conditions associated with an increased risk of embolic stroke include marantic endocarditis, Libman–Sacks endocarditis due to systemic lupus erythematosus with antiphospholipid antibodies and calcification of the mitral annulus. Patients who have aortic plaques >4 mm in thickness at TEE have a high risk of stroke, and some of these events may be embolic[33].

The results of several major randomized trials of anticoagulation in primary and secondary prevention of stroke in patients with non-rheumatic atrial fibrillation have been reported during the last decade and have transformed clinical practice[34–39]. Without anticoagulant treatment, 5–8% of patients >60 years of age with atrial fibrillation showed evidence of an ischemic brain event every year.

Warfarin anticoagulation to achieve an international normalized ratio of between 1.5 and 4.0 reduces the risk by around 20% with less than 2.5% of significant bleeding events per year. Aspirin is apparently somewhat less effective, but still confers benefit compared with no treatment. It is still important to recognize that indiscriminate use of warfarin in elderly patients with atrial fibrillation may cause bleeding complications. For this reason, some of the trials used rigorous exclusion criteria so that only a relatively small proportion of patients with atrial fibrillation were admitted.

Younger patients with lone atrial fibrillation appear to have a low risk of stroke. Not surprisingly, previous stroke or TIA, fibrillation, recent heart failure or a history of hypertension defines groups with a relatively high risk of embolic events.

The optimal level of anticoagulation for secondary prevention in non-rheumatic atrial fibrillation appears to be at an international normalized ratio of 3.0[40]. All patients >60 years of age should receive antithrombotic treatment unless there is a definite contraindication.

In the first 2 weeks following myocardial infarction, 1–5% of patients have an ischemic stroke. The risk is particularly high after anterior events and if there are areas of dyskinesia[41]. Full anticoagulation with heparin prevents ischemic events after anterior infarction, and aspirin treatment reduces the incidence. The combination of low-dose heparin with aspirin appears to reduce the risk of ischemic stroke to 1% or less shortly after infarction, although full-dose heparin treatment is generally preferred.

Thrombolytic treatment alone apparently does not have much effect on the frequency of ischemic stroke caused by mural thrombus. An appreciable risk of embolism (around 10% per year) is found in patients with continuing evidence of ventricular thrombus. In these patients, low-intensity anticoagulation with warfarin is the best treatment.

An important unresolved difficulty in the treatment of patients with cardiogenic embolic stroke is the optimal timing and nature of anticoagulant therapy. The risk of hemorrhagic transformation of large cerebral infarcts is high, and will most likely become visible on CT between 12h and 4 days after onset.

Anticoagulation increases the risk of late hemorrhage, which may result in deterioration of neurological status. The current practice is to defer anticoagulant treatment for a variable period of up to 10 days in high-risk patients with large infarcts, but there is an urgent need for clinical trials to inform practice. Any risk of immediate hemorrhagic transformation has to be balanced against the risk of further embolism, which appears to be approximately 10% over 2 weeks, although there is wide variation across series.

Mode of onset is sometimes helpful in determining other causes of ischemic stroke. The classical stuttering onset occurs in a small proportion of atherothrombotic events and, in some cases, lacunar strokes may show a slow progressive worsening of symptoms over 24–48h.

Headache after cerebral infarction may indicate embolism, but the degree of discrimination is low as up to 30% of patients with ischemic stroke have headache. The peak incidence of ischemic stroke, as with hemorrhage, is between 0800h and 1000h, a period when arterial pressures tend to be high. A potential confounding factor in these analyses is the inclusion of individuals whose onset of stroke is some time before awakening.

Unfortunately, CT is of limited value in the diagnosis of early ischemic stroke, and changes are often undetectable or subtle in the early hours. Full delineation of the area of infarction is best after 7–10 days. The newer-generation scanners are better able to detect the early changes of infarction, such as effacement of the distinction between white and gray matter, and blurring of the normal sulcal patterns. Periods of isodensity occurring around 3 days after infarction occasionally cause difficulties. Infarcts in the brain stem tend to be poorly visualized, but those in the cerebellar hemispheres are reasonably well-defined.

MRI, and T_2-weighted scans in particular, are better able to localize brain-stem ischemic events and small deep infarcts or lacunar infarcts. Contrast enhancement with gadolinium increases sensitivity, but may give false-positive results.

Ischemic changes can be seen on T_2-weighted MRI early in the development of ischemic stroke but, at this stage, MRI is less reliable in differentiating hemorrhage from infarction. The suggestion that SPECT may be a better predictor of outcome than clinical scoring has yet to be confirmed.

The extent of cerebral infarction varies widely among subjects even when the same artery has been occluded. Internal carotid artery occlusion may cause devastating hemispheric infarction in some patients, but only a TIA, or no symptoms at all, in others.

The extent of infarction after carotid or middle cerebral artery occlusion clearly depends on the adequacy of the collaterals. The size of the posterior communicating artery on the relevant side has been identified as an important determinant of the extent of infarction. The collateral circulation established during a preexisting period of arterial stenosis may also be important.

In contrast to findings in white Europeans, occlusion of the middle cerebral artery stem is a relatively common cause of atherosclerotic stroke in Eastern Asia and Africa. The result is widespread subcortical infarction in the territories of the lenticulostriate and other perforating arteries, with or without major infarction of the superficial middle cerebral artery territory.

In rats with experimentally induced middle cerebral artery occlusion, the extent of infarction is apparently much greater in animals with certain genetic strains of hypertension, but the determinants of this susceptibility have not yet been ascertained. It is fairly certain that structural changes in cerebral arteries as a result of hypertension limit collateral blood flow after vascular occlusion.

The stress of major stroke often increases plasma concentrations of glucose, and high plasma glucose levels appear to have an adverse effect on infarct size and prognosis. Blood pressures are commonly raised immediately post-stroke, with loss of the usual nocturnal dip. However, the safety of anti-hypertensive therapy during this phase, when autoregulatory mechanisms are improved, is not established.

Care in an acute stroke unit compared with a general medical ward has been shown to reduce mortality and improve functional outcome[42–45]. The individual components of care have not been identified, but maintenance of an airway, proper assessment of swallowing, and better management of fluid and glucose metabolism are likely to be involved. It is estimated that the minimum increase in staff in a general ward compared with a dedicated stroke unit is 1.0 for the number of nurses, and 0.3 each for physiotherapists and occupational therapists, for every six patients.

Lacunar stroke

Small infarcts deep in the cerebral hemispheres and in the brain stem caused by occlusion of perforating end arteries originating in the circle of Willis, and of the proximal middle, posterior cerebral and basilar arteries, are often described as 'lacunar'. The term derives from gross pathology where a lacune refers to a small slit-like space usually in the basal ganglia or basis pontis. The typical appearance of lacunar strokes may be the result of areas of infarction that are 2–15 mm in diameter, but resorption of small areas of hemorrhage may produce an identical appearance. Lacunes may develop silently in many instances.

A number of well-defined stroke syndromes – termed lacunar syndromes – are believed to result from occlusion of a single penetrating artery causing infarcts that are 0.5–2 cm in diameter. Approximately 10–20% of strokes in Europe and in the USA are lacunar syndromes.

Historically, this type of stroke was linked causally to hypertensive small-vessel disease, although some doubt has been cast on this simple concept. The syndrome may be caused by atherosclerosis. C. Miller Fisher originally described a type of medial degeneration in affected vessels which he termed 'lipohyalinosis', but the pathological process leading to most of the small-vessel occlusion remains under dispute. Furthermore, the relationship to the more familiar larger-artery atherosclerosis remains poorly defined.

The most commonly encountered lacunar syndrome is pure motor hemiplegia, affecting the face, arm and leg, as a result of infarction in the internal capsule or in the basis pontis. In some cases, infarction is situated in the corona radiata, cerebral peduncle or, less commonly, medulla oblongata. A relatively high proportion of these small deep infarcts are not visualized on CT, which creates further difficulties in making accurate neuroanatomical correlations. MRI has greater sensitivity, but may produce a high proportion of false-positive results, and may not allow differentiation between infarction and areas of demyelination caused by other processes.

The clinical definition of the lacunar syndromes is dependent on the proximity of motor fibers to the face, arm and leg within the relevant areas of white matter and especially the posterior internal capsule. A proportion of patients with partial syndromes, and especially with weakness confined to the arm and leg, have small deep infarcts. However, expanding the definition to include patients with brachiofacial weakness will significantly increase the proportion of patients in whom cortical infarcts are found.

By definition, aphasia, visuospatial neglect, agnosia, apraxia and visual-field deficits do not occur in lacunar syndromes, but may be present as a result of larger striatocapsular infarcts, which probably have a different etiology. In comparison to hemiplegia caused by cortical infarcts, pure motor hemiplegia due to small deep infarcts carries a considerably better prognosis in terms of recovery of functional capacity.

Pure sensory stroke is another lacunar syndrome that accounts for <10% of all clinical lacunar syndromes. They are caused by very small infarcts in the thalamus, the bulk of which is supplied by branches of the posterior cerebral artery, except for the anterior pole. Clinically, patients often present with symptoms of widespread unilateral paresthesia and, on occasions, there is an element of dissociated sensory loss. Pure sensory stroke may evolve after several months into a distressing syndrome of chronic pain in the affected side.

The original concept of lacunar infarction did not include sensorimotor stroke because of the separate blood supplies to the thalamus and posterior internal capsule. However, it is now clear that such strokes can be caused by small deep infarcts. Diagnostic precision in terms of locating sensorimotor strokes is not as accurate as with either pure motor or pure sensory strokes.

Other classical lacunar syndromes are homolateral ataxia, and crural paresis and dysarthria with clumsy hand, both of which may be encompassed in the term 'ataxic hemiparesis' and may be caused by small infarcts in the basis pontis. The syndrome is not common, and dysmetria may be difficult to detect clinically in a weak limb. Some small brainstem infarcts with a central location may be caused by small-vessel disease, but clinical definition is difficult. Warning TIAs quite often occur before the definitive event in lacunar stroke.

Clinical distinction of lacunar infarcts from small deep hemorrhages is rarely possible without CT. As hypertensive cerebral hemorrhage and lacunar infarction both originate in small deep perforators, a common etiological mechanism is likely. Because lacunar infarcts are small, deep and distant from pain-sensitive tissues, headache is unusual.

Intracerebral hemorrhage

Bleeding into the brain as a cause of acute stroke was described in as early as the sixteenth and seventeenth centuries, but the burgeoning pathological description in the nineteenth century firmly defined hemorrhage as a cause of stroke. Charcot and Duret dubbed the lateral lenticulostriate artery the 'artery of cerebral hemorrhage'. Bouchard and Charcot recognized the origin of bleeding from microaneurysms as early as 1868 at virtually the same time that Mohamed at Guy's Hospital in London began to recognize clinical hypertension.

A completely reliable distinction of hemorrhage from infarction in patients was not possible until the development of CT in the early 1970s. In the acute situation, CT is unrivalled as a method of diagnosis although MRI, which is able to detect hemosiderin, is more useful than CT in the chronic stage. Contrast angiography is only necessary to define aneurysms and vascular malformation.

Hematomas commonly increase in size in the hour or two after admission and may continue to increase for 12 h or longer. Deeply placed hematomas, especially in the putamen, are characteristic of hypertension. Not surprisingly, most episodes of bleeding start at times of the day when arterial pressures are high. This is also the case with subarachnoid hemorrhage due to aneurysm rupture.

In recent years, a novel pathology has been shown to cause more superficial or lobar cerebral hemorrhages, events which may account for more than 50% of bleeds in Europe and North America, and a high proportion of events in the elderly. Many are now known to be caused by rupture of vessels with amyloid deposits in the walls[46]. Amyloid shows a predilection for the cortical veins, arteries and vessels of the leptomeninges. Hemorrhage caused by amyloid angiopathy is increasingly common in patients aged 60 years and over. Bleeding is often initiated at the junction of gray and white matter.

Amyloid deposition tends to spare vessels supplying the basal ganglia and brain stem, although it may be present in the vessels of the cerebellar hemispheres. Bleeding is sometimes multicentric and, in some instances, premonitory symptoms resembling TIAs have been described. These symptoms may be due to areas of ischemia and infarction, or to minute areas of hemorrhage triggering waves of spreading depression, as in migraine. When amyloid angiopathy is the cause of cerebral hemorrhage, recurrence is likely.

Other causes of lobar hemorrhage include vascular malformations and some metastatic cerebral tumors, malignant melanoma in particular, and abuse of sympathomimetic drugs such as cocaine.

Overtreatment with anticoagulants may present similarly, and there is some evidence that bleeding after thrombolytic treatment of myocardial infarction may be predominantly lobar. The safety of thrombolytic therapy for acute stroke with symptoms for > 3h has not been established. The average risk of intracerebral hemorrhage in treated patients is around 10%, or three-and-one-half times that of controls[47].

The clinical symptoms of lobar hemorrhage, but not deep hemorrhage, are headache and early seizure accompanied by few signs of chronic hypertension. Vomiting is a powerful predictor of hemorrhage in supratentorial stroke; it occurs especially in cases of hemorrhage into the caudate nucleus. Proximity of the caudate nucleus to the ventricular system predisposes to rupture into the lateral ventricles, which leads to an abrupt increase in intracranial pressure. Blood pressures after intracerebral hemorrhage tend to be higher than after cerebral infarction.

Hypertensive cerebral hemorrhage most often originates in the putamen. The classical findings in large putaminal hemorrhages are hemiplegia, hemisensory loss, hemianopia, conjugate deviation of the eyes towards the side of the lesion, impaired consciousness, aphasia or contralateral neglect depending on hemispheric dominance. Hyperreflexia may be present at an early stage. Smaller anterior and posterior lesions tend to have a better prognosis than those located more centrally, but coma carries a very poor prognosis.

Thalamic hemorrhage with pressure on the midbrain tends to cause abnormalities of vertical gaze wherein the eyes are deviated downwards and inwards. Sensory deficits are prominent and transcortical sensory aphasias may occur. Hypersomnolence may result from local pressure on the reticular activating system of the rostral brain stem.

Cerebellar hemorrhage presents with headache, vertigo, vomiting and an inability to stand, and compression of the pons often causes peripheral facial weakness and horizontal gaze palsy. Gait and truncal ataxia, and ipsilateral limb ataxia, may be difficult to recognize in the acute phase. Hemorrhage into the pons almost always causes a reduced level of consciousness. Bilateral gaze paresis and quadriplegia are often present.

A uniform finding after intracerebral hemorrhage is that the prognosis is best predicted by the level of consciousness at presentation. This has led to widespread clinical application of numerical systems that grade severity, such as the widely used Glasgow Coma Scale. Not surprisingly, the volume of hematoma in supratentorial events is a predictor of survival and potential outcome. The amount of blood in the ventricular system is another factor of prognostic significance. The overall rate of mortality at 30 days is 35–50%.

The role of surgical evacuation in treatment is still a matter of dispute, and there are few randomized controlled trials to inform clinical practice. Operations tend to be carried out on less severely affected patients, and those with lobar and cerebellar hemorrhage fare better than those with bleeding centered on the basal ganglia. Small-scale trials of surgical treatment of putaminal hemorrhage have arrived at different conclusions.

Newer surgical techniques, mostly pioneered in Japan, include stereostatic drainage under CT guidance occasionally supplemented by aspiration after instillation of fibrinolytics. Here again, the younger and less severely affected patients appear to have the better outcomes. It is clear that large-scale randomized controlled trials need to be carried out to clarify the situation.

Vascular causes of dementia

The prevalence of vascular dementia is difficult to determine because the criteria for diagnosis are imprecise and vary widely. However, there is general agreement that vascular causes are most likely in patients aged 85 years or older. Recently, there has been a growing awareness that the most frequent vascular cause of dementia is white-matter ischemia and not multiple cerebral infarctions. Although Alzheimer's disease is undoubtedly the most common dementing process, it is not clear at present whether vascular disease or Lewy body dementia is the more frequent. Clinical dementia may be caused by a multi-infarct state, but the neuropathology is often complicated by the presence of more than one disease process. Histopathological studies have variously concluded that vascular factors may be involved in 10–40% of cases.

Clinical evidence of multiple infarcts may be adduced from mode of onset, fluctuating deficits, focal neurological symptoms and signs of emotional lability. With cerebral infarction, the site may be as important as the volume of brain lost. Multiple cortical infarcts caused by cardiogenic embolism may cause dementia; the most commonly seen clinical findings in these cases are aphasia, agnosia, apraxia and memory loss.

One infarct in a critical area may also cause dementia without multiple events[48]. Infarction of the angular gyrus in the inferior parietal lobule, for example, may cause dementia accompanied by Wernicke's aphasia, with or without right, left and finger agnosias, acalculia, agraphia and visuospatial abnormalities. Stroke in the ventromedial sector of the frontal lobes may have devastating effects on behavior by causing apathy and an inability to initiate either activity or conversation. Bilateral infarction of both caudate nuclei has similar effects.

Subcortical lacunar events causing dementia are characterized by psychomotor retardation and abulia combined with a shuffling gait (*marche à petit pas*), bilateral spasticity, dysphagia, dysarthria and emotional incontinence. Hypertension has been predictive of white-matter lesions on MRI in population surveys[49].

A rare genetic syndrome termed CADASIL (cerebral autosomal-dominant arteriopathy with subcortical infarcts and leukoencephalopathy) has recently been described in a number of European families with reported linkage to chromosome 19. Recurrent ischemic symptoms start at a relatively young age, and progress to pseudobulbar palsy and subcortical dementia, with death tending to occur within 10 years of presentation. MRI reveals a marked increase in signal intensity from subcortical white matter with multiple small deep infarcts, but sparing of the cerebral cortex.

The advent of modalities such as CT and especially MRI has drawn attention to the frequent occurrence of white-matter lesions in elderly patients. Periventricular low attenuation on CT, also referred to as leukoariosis, is common with advancing age, and probably represents demyelination and gliosis as a consequence of arteriosclerosis of the long penetrating end arterioles. The cerebral cortex presumably becomes disconnected as a consequence.

In a report by Longstreth and colleagues of a large population-based MRI study of cardiovascular health in elderly subjects[50], high-grade white-matter lesions were more often found in patients who presented with gait problems and cognitive decline. These results support the original concept of Binswanger's disease as being caused by chronic ischemia of the end arteries of the medulla.

The Cardiovascular Health Study has also shed light on the vexed question of the significance of so-called unidentified bright objects (UBOs). Punctate bilateral UBOs appear to correspond to dilated perivascular spaces around spirally elongated penetrating arteries. Lacunar infarcts in the basal ganglia, internal capsule, pons, thalamus and centrum ovale were also frequent findings.

Another finding of this study was that white-matter disease was more likely to be seen in patients with hypertension and vascular risk factors such as cigarette-smoking. Surprisingly, diabetes mellitus did not appear to be predictive of lesions. Follow-up studies in this cohort are likely to resolve many of the questions regarding the clinical significance of white-matter lesions seen on MRI.

Stroke prevention

The ultimate goal of all stroke interventions is to prevent death and disability from stroke. Stroke prevention strategies may occur at multiple stages: in the healthy, stroke-free, population (primary prevention); among those who have developed recognizable risk factors and who may have subclinical disease (late primary or early secondary prevention); and after the development of neurological symptoms of stroke or TIAs (late secondary or tertiary prevention). Despite the excitement surrounding acute therapies, there still remains a significant challenge to prove that pharmacological agents deemed successful in animal studies are able to reduce the burden of stroke hours after the initial injury has occurred. Further emphasis needs to be placed on the advances that have been made in the ability to detect who is at increased risk of stroke and to then modify this risk whenever possible to prevent stroke before it is too late to reverse its consequences.

Some stroke risk factors are not modifiable whereas others are easily amenable to modification by medical or surgical intervention (see Section 2, Figure 4[51]). Although cerebrovascular disorders may occur at any age, at any time, in either sex, in all races and regardless of family history, each of these non-modifiable factors has an effect on the incidence of stroke.

Age is the strongest determinant of stroke and, as the population ages, the number of strokes is projected to greatly increase. Men usually have a greater incidence of stroke than women, but the greater life expectancy among women leads to a greater stroke prevalence for women. Certain race–ethnic groups, such as African–Americans and Hispanics, have an increased incidence of stroke, and the changing demographic profiles in the USA may also contribute to the greater number of strokes being predicted in the coming years[52,53]. Genetic factors are now being identified as potential determinants of stroke risk, and novel insights into genetic–environmental interactions may change the current approach to stroke prevention. At present, however, non-modifiable factors or risk markers serve best to alert clinicians to potential high-risk groups and to encourage a more diligent approach to treating modifiable risk factors.

The major modifiable risk factors for stroke include hypertension, cardiac disease (particularly atrial fibrillation), diabetes, dyslipidemia, cigarette-smoking and alcohol abuse, physical inactivity and asymptomatic carotid stenosis. Epidemiological studies have shown that each of these conditions elevates the risk of stroke, and randomized clinical trials in certain circumstances have provided definitive indications as to the best therapy to prevent stroke. The public-health impact of these conditions depends upon the relative risk or odds ratio, which is a measure of potency, and the prevalence, which is a measure of how frequently the condition is found in the general population. Stroke prevention campaigns usually concentrate on those conditions that have moderate relative risks, a greater prevalence, and readily available and effective treatments.

Hypertension

After age, hypertension is the most important determinant of stroke. The risk of stroke rises proportionately with elevated diastolic and systolic blood pressures. In a multivariate model from the Framingham Study[54], the relative risk of stroke for an increase of 10 mmHg in systolic blood pressure was 1.9 for men and 1.7 for women, after controlling for other known stroke risk factors. Isolated systolic hypertension and borderline elevated blood pressures within the range generally considered normotensive also increase the risk of stroke[55]. What makes hypertension even more important is its high prevalence in both men and women, and its especially high prevalence in certain race–ethnic groups. The proportion of strokes attributable to hypertension is 50–60%.

Prospective studies and clinical trials have consistently shown a decreased risk of stroke with control of mild, moderate and severe hypertension in all age groups. Meta-analysis of nine prospective studies involving 420 000 subjects followed for 10 years found that stroke risk increased by 46% for every 7.5-mmHg increase in diastolic blood pressure[56]. Meta-analysis of 14 treatment trials involving 50 000 participants followed for a mean of 5 years demonstrated a substantial reduction in stroke risk. The analysis showed a mean diastolic reduction of 5–6 mmHg to correspond to a 35–40% reduction in all or fatal strokes[57].

Moreover, clinical trials have demonstrated significant benefits for the treatment of hypertension in the elderly, even among those with isolated systolic hypertension[58,59]. Finally, some community-based hypertension treatment-control programs, designed to detect, treat and monitor hypertensive patients of all ages by integrating patient education and training of healthcare personnel, have documented a successful reduction in stroke[60]. More effective control of hypertension could have a major impact on reducing the public health burden of stroke. In the USA, it has been estimated that 246 500 strokes could be prevented by control of hypertension alone, which would result in a savings of 12.33 billion dollars[61].

Cardiac conditions

Various cardiac conditions have been shown to increase the risk of ischemic stroke. Some cardiac conditions may be viewed as intervening events in the causal chain of stroke because certain risk factors, such as hypertension, are also determinants of cardiac disease. Most studies, however, have indicated that conditions such as atrial fibrillation, valvular heart disease, myocardial infarction (MI), coronary artery disease, congestive heart failure and electrocardiographic evidence of left ventricular hypertrophy are independent predictors of stroke. New information is being accumulated regarding the importance of patent foramen ovale, atrial septal aneurysm, mitral valve strands and aortic arch atheroma as risk factors for stroke.

Atrial fibrillation

Chronic atrial fibrillation is a potent predictor of stroke. In the Framingham Study, the risk of stroke was increased nearly 20-fold when atrial fibrillation was associated with valvular disease, and nearly fivefold with non-valvular atrial fibrillation[62]. It has been estimated that atrial fibrillation affects more than 2 000 000 Americans and becomes more frequent with age, ranking as the leading cardiac arrhythmia in the elderly. Therefore, the proportion of strokes attributable to atrial fibrillation increases significantly with age, approaching that of hypertension among those ages 80–89 years.

Multiple randomized clinical trials have demonstrated the superior therapeutic effects of warfarin, which has an international normalized ratio (INR) of 2.0–3.0, compared with placebo and compared with aspirin in the prevention of thromboembolic events among asymptomatic patients with nonvalvular atrial fibrillation[34–38,63,64]. The role of aspirin in the prevention of stroke with atrial fibrillation was also established by the modest risk reduction with 325 mg of aspirin *vs* placebo in the Stroke Prevention in Atrial Fibrillation (SPAF I) trial[38]. The recommendation of the Fifth American College of Chest Physicians Consensus Conference on Antithrombotic Therapy was that '...long-term oral anticoagulant therapy (target INR 2.5; range 2.0–3.0) be considered for all AF patients who are at high risk of stroke'[65].

Other cardiac conditions

For other cardiac conditions, the stroke risk nearly doubles in those with antecedent coronary artery disease, trebles with left ventricular hypertrophy and nearly quadruples in patients with cardiac failure[51]. Acute MI has been associated with stroke, particularly when it is transmural or involves the anterior wall. Uncomplicated angina, non-Q-wave infarction and silent MI have all been found to indicate increased risk of stroke. Mitral stenosis, endocarditis and prosthetic heart valves are only some of the valvular diseases that increase the risk of stroke.

Measures that are effective in reducing the incidence of cardiac disease might lead to a reduction in stroke incidence, although the clinical trial evidence supporting this claim is lacking. Antiplate-let agents have proved efficacious in the reduction of non-fatal MI in primary prevention studies among US and UK physicians, but have not been shown to significantly reduce stroke in such low-risk populations[66,67]. Warfarin appears to be beneficial in the prevention of cardiogenic embolism among patients with acute anterior wall MI, left atrial or ventricular thrombus and prosthetic valve replacements. The effectiveness of anticoagulation in reducing stroke in the setting of congestive heart failure remains controversial and unproven in randomized trials.

Diabetes mellitus

Diabetes mellitus is a risk factor for ischemic stroke, and increases the risk of atherosclerosis and microangiopathy of the coronary, peripheral and cerebral arteries. Studies have demonstrated an independent effect of diabetes, with a relative risk ranging from 1.5–3.0 even after other stroke risk factors have been controlled for[68,69]. Diabetes is frequently associated with small-vessel ischemic or 'lacunar' infarction. Although there is a paucity of clinical trial data on the effects of diabetes treatment on the risk of stroke, there is evidence to indicate that tight glycemic control results in a reduction in other diabetic complications[70]. Clinical wisdom suggests that better control of diabetes would translate into reduced stroke risk.

Lipids

Triglyceride, cholesterol, low-density lipoprotein (LDL) and high-density lipoprotein (HDL) have a more definitive relationship to atherosclerosis and coronary artery disease than to cerebrovascular disease[71]. The inconsistent results reported in studies regarding the relationship between cholesterol and stroke have been partly due to the heterogeneity of stroke subtypes of which, primarily, those due to atherosclerosis may be related to blood lipids, the later age of onset and lower incidence of stroke compared with heart disease. Studies of extracranial carotid atherosclerosis, however, have demonstrated that the degree and progression of plaque are directly related to cholesterol and LDL, and inversely related to HDL[72]. Finally, impressive evidence has been documented in randomized clinical trials that carotid plaque can regress in – and ischemic stroke outcomes be reduced among – those patients treated with the latest generation of cholesterol-lowering agents[73].

Cigarette-smoking

This is a major public health problem, given the estimates that nearly 410 000 Americans die each year from causes attributed to cigarette-smoking. Epidemiological studies have consistently shown a significant effect of smoking on stroke: a pooled adjusted relative risk of 1.5; a dose–response relationship with increased stroke risks for heavier smokers; and reductions in stroke risk among those who quit smoking[74,75]. Cigarette-smoking is known to be an independent determinant of carotid artery plaque thickness and the strongest predictor of severe extracranial carotid artery atherosclerosis[76].

In addition to inducing atherosclerosis, cigarette-smoking promotes stroke by increasing blood viscosity, coagulability, fibrinogen levels, platelet aggregation and pressure. In the USA, it is estimated that 61 000 strokes could be prevented annually by controlling smoking, with an associated savings of more than 3 billion dollars per year. The health risks from continued cigarette-smoking are unquestionable and the message that quitting at any time reduces the risk of stroke unequivocal.

Alcohol consumption

Whether there is also a causal relationship between alcohol intake and stroke remains controversial; the correlation is most likely dose-dependent. The results of epidemiological studies have ranged from demonstrating a definite independent effect in both men and women to indicating an effect only in men and showing no effect after controlling for other confounding risk factors such as cigarette-smoking[77]. Chronic heavy drinking and acute intoxication have been associated with both hemorrhagic and ischemic stroke. The mechanisms through which alcohol increases the risk of stroke include the promotion of hypertension, hypercoagulable states, cardiac arrhythmias and cerebral blood flow reduction. Alternatively, there is evidence that light-to-moderate drinking can increase HDL cholesterol and reduce the risk of coronary artery disease. This protective association has been corroborated by the demonstration of a J-shaped relationship between alcohol intake and ischemic stroke, an elevated ischemic stroke risk with heavy alcohol consumption and a protective effect among light-to-moderate drinkers compared with non-drinkers[78].

Physical activity

This has been recognized as having beneficial cardiovascular effects. There is now accumulated evidence that stroke risks are also reduced among those who are physically active[79,80]. In the Northern Manhattan Stroke Study[81], leisure-time physical activity was found to be significantly associated with a reduced risk of stroke among men and women, young and old, and whites, blacks and Hispanics. A full 25% of the stroke-free population reported no physical activity in the 2 weeks prior to the interview, suggesting that lack of physical activity is an important modifiable risk factor. Although the study found a dose–response relationship indicating that heavier activity and longer duration of activity were more beneficial, light activities such as walking, in which even the most elderly individuals can engage, conferred a significant protective effect. The US Centers for Disease Control have recommended that all

Americans undertake at least 30 min of moderately intense physical activity on most, and preferably all, days of the week[82].

Asymptomatic carotid artery stenosis

This determinant of ischemic stroke confers annual risks of 2.5% for vascular events, 3.3% for ipsilateral stroke and 10.5% for TIAs or stroke among those with >75% stenosis[83]. Moreover, the prevalence of carotid stenosis increases with age. The development of cerebral ischemia probably depends on the degree and progression of the carotid stenosis, sufficiency of collateral circulation, constitution of the atherosclerotic plaque and propensity to form thrombus at the site of stenosis.

The role of prophylactic endarterectomy in those with asymptomatic extracranial carotid artery stenosis is somewhat controversial. The ACAS trial demonstrated a statistical benefit for carotid endarterectomy for those with stenosis of ≥60%[19]. Among the 1662 patients randomized to either carotid endarterectomy and best medical therapy *vs* best medical therapy alone (aspirin 325 mg daily plus risk-factor modification), the 5-year risk of ipsilateral stroke was 11% in the medical group and 5.1% in the surgical group (a 53% relative-risk reduction). Any decision regarding the use of endarterectomy for asymptomatic carotid stenosis patients should depend on minimizing the potential complications by selecting patients who are good surgical candidates with stable or no cardiac disease and by using an experienced surgeon to maintain an operative stroke risk of <3%.

Prevention of recurrent stroke

When a patient develops symptoms of cerebral ischemia and presents with a TIA or cerebral infarction, there are options from which to choose for the prevention of first or recurrent stroke, depending on the mechanism of the event. For those who have symptomatic significant carotid stenosis, carotid endarterectomy is of indisputable value[16–18]. For those with a definite source of cardiac embolism, oral anticoagulation has been demonstrated to be effective in the prevention of cardioembolic stroke[39]. For patients with other causes of cerebral ischemia, a variety of antiplatelet agents have proved to be of value in the prevention of ischemic stroke, including aspirin, extended-release dipyridamole plus aspirin, clopidogrel and ticlopidine[21–24]. New antiplatelet agents are currently being tested in a variety of circumstances among patients with cerebrovascular disorders.

Conclusions

Stroke prevention requires identification of those subjects at an increased risk of stroke, modification of risk factors where possible, and institution of treatments among patients who have already developed TIAs or stroke. Our understanding of the risk factors for stroke and the potential ways to modify them continues to grow at a rapid pace. In addition, clinical trials have shown that antihypertensive agents, antiplatelet drugs, warfarin, certain lipid-lowering compounds and surgery may reduce stroke risk in appropriately selected patients.

In the absence of a 'miracle drug' that reverses acute ischemic stroke, the most promising approach to reduce the future burden of ischemic stroke is to more effectively practice stroke prevention.

References

1. Malmgren R, Warlow C, Sandercock P, Slattery P. Geographical and secular trends in stroke incidence. *Lancet* 1987;ii:1196–1200

2. Bonita R, Stewart A, Beaglehole R. International trends in stroke mortalities: 1970–1985. *Stroke* 1990;21:989–92

3. Bonita R. Epidemiological studies and the prevention of stroke. *Cerebrovasc Dis* 1994;4 (Suppl 1):2–10

4. Eisenblätter D, Heinemann L, Classen E. Community-based stroke incidence trends from the 1970s through the 1980s in East Germany. *Stroke* 1995;26:919–23

5. Brown RD, Whisnant JP, Sicks JD, O'Fallon WM, Wiebers DO. Stroke incidence, prevalence and survival. *Stroke* 1996;27:373–80

6. American Heart Association. *1998 Heart and Stroke Facts*. Dallas: AHA, 1997

7. National Stroke Association. *Brain Attack Briefing Update*. Denver: NSA, 1998

8. Bamford J, Sandercock P, Dennis M, Burn J, Warlow C. Classification and national history of clinically identifiable subtypes of cerebral infarction. *Lancet* 1991;337:1521–6

9. Fisher CM. Lacunar infarcts – A review. *Cerebrovasc Dis* 1991;1:311–20

10. Foulkes MA, Wolf PA, Price TR, *et al*. The Stroke Data Bank: Design, methods, and baseline characteristics. *Stroke* 1998;19:547–54

11. National Institute of Neurological Diseases and Stroke. Classification of cerebrovascular diseases. III. *Stroke* 1990;21:637–76

12. Chen J, Simon R. Ischaemic tolerance in the brain. *Neurology* 1997;48:306–11

13. Ringelstein EB. Skepticism toward carotid ultrasonography: A virtue, an attitude or fanaticism. *Stroke* 1995;26:1743–6

14. Alexandrov AV, Bladin CF, Maggisano R, Norris JW. Measuring carotid stenosis: Time for a reappraisal. *Stroke* 1993;24:1292–6

15. Wilterdink JL, Feldmann F, Easton D, Ward R. Performance of carotid ultrasound in evaluating candidates for carotid endarterectomy is optimized by an approach based on clinical outcome rather than accuracy. *Stroke* 1996; 27:1094–8

16. European Carotid Surgery Trialists' Collaborative Group. Randomised trial of endarterectomy for recently symptomatic carotid stenosis: Final results of the MRC European Carotid Surgery Trial (ECST). *Lancet* 1998;351:1379–87

17. North American Symptomatic Carotid Endarterectomy Trial Collaborators. Beneficial effect of carotid endarterectomy in symptomatic patients with high-grade carotid stenosis. *N Engl J Med* 1991; 325:445–53

18. Mayberg MR, Wilson SE, Yatsu F, *et al.* Carotid endarterectomy and prevention of cerebral ischemia in symptomatic carotid stenosis: Veterans Affairs Cooperative Studies Program 309 Trialist Group. *JAMA* 1991;266:3289–44

19. Executive Committee for the Asymptomatic Carotid Atherosclerosis Study. Endarterectomy for asymptomatic carotid artery stenosis. *JAMA* 1995;273:1421–8

20. Paddock-Eliasziw LM, Eliasziw M, Barr HWK, *et al.* Long-term prognosis and the effect of carotid endarterectomy in patients with ipsilateral ischaemic events. *Neurology* 1996;47: 1158–62

21. Antiplatelet Trialists' Collaboration. Collaborative overview of randomised trials of antiplatelet therapy. 1: Prevention of death, myocardial therapy in various categories of patients. *Br Med J* 1994;308:81–106

22. CAPRIE Steering Committee. A randomised, blinded, trial of clopidogrel versus aspirin in patients at risk of ischaemic events (CAPRIE). *Lancet* 1996;348:1329–39

23. Diener HC, Cunha L, Forbes C, *et al.* European Stroke Prevention Study 2: Dipyridamole and acetylsalicylic acid in the secondary prevention of stroke. *J Neurol Sci* 1996;143:1–13

24. Hart RG, Harrison MJG. Aspirin wars. The optimal dose of aspirin to prevent stroke. *Stroke* 1996;27:585–7

25. Barnett HJM, Kaste M, Meldrum H, Eliasziw M. Aspirin dose in stroke prevention. Beautiful hypothesis slain by ugly facts. *Stroke* 1996;27: 588–92

26. Cerebral Embolism Task Force. Cardiogenic brain embolism: Second report of the Cerebral Embolism Task Force. *Arch Neurol* 1989;46: 727–41

27. Bogousslavsky J, Cachin C, Regli F, *et al.* Cardiac sources of embolism and cerebral infarction: Clinical consequences and vascular concomitants. *Neurology* 1991;41:855–9

28. Loh E, Sutton M St J, Wun C-CC, *et al.* Ventricular dysfunction and the risk of stroke after myocardial infarction. *N Engl J Med* 1997; 336:251–7

29. Sandercock PAG, Warlow CP, Jones LN, Starkey IR. Predisposing factors for cerebral infarction: The Oxfordshire Community Stroke Project. *Br Med J* 1989;298:75–80

30. Turpie AGG, Gent M, Laupacis A, *et al.* A comparison of aspirin with placebo in patients treated with warfarin after heart valve replacement. *N Engl J Med* 1993;19:524–9

31. Lechat P, Mas JL, Lascault G, *et al.* Prevalence of patent foramen ovale in patients with stroke. *N Engl J Med* 1988;318:1148–52

32. Jauss M, Kaps M, Keberle M, Haberbosch W, Dorndorf W. A comparison of transesophageal echocardiography and transcranial Doppler sonography with contrast medium for detection of patent foramen ovale. *Stroke* 1994;25:1265–7

33. The French Study of Aortic Plaques in Stroke Groups. Atherosclerotic disease of the aortic arch as a risk factor for recurrent ischemic stroke. *N Engl J Med* 1996;334:1216–21

34. The Boston Area Anticoagulation Trial for Atrial Fibrillation Investigators. The effect of low-dose warfarin on the risk of stroke in patients with non-rheumatic atrial fibrillation. *N Engl J Med* 1990;323:1505–11

35. Connolly SJ, Laupacis A, Gent M, Roberts RS, Cairns JA, Joyner C. Canadian Atrial Fibrillation Anticoagulation (CAFA) Study. *J Am Coll Cardiol* 1991;18:349–55

36. Ezekowitz MD, Bridgers SL, James KE, *et al.* Warfarin in the prevention of stroke associated with nonrheumatic atrial fibrillation. *N Engl J Med* 1992;327:1406–12 (Erratum *N Engl J Med* 1993; 328:148)

37. Peterson P, Godtfredson J, Anderson B, Boysen G, Anderson ED. Placebo-controlled, randomised trial of warfarin and aspirin for prevention of thromboembolic complications in chronic atrial fibrillation: The Copenhagen AFASAK Study. *Lancet* 1989;i:175–9

38. McBride R. Stroke Prevention in Atrial Fibrillation Study: Final results. *Circulation* 1991;84: 527–39

39. EAFT (European Atrial Fibrillation Trial) Study Group. Secondary prevention in non-rheumatic atrial fibrillation after transient ischaemic attack in minor stroke. *Lancet* 1993;342:1255–62

40. European and Atrial Fibrillation Trial Study Groups. Optimal anticoagulant therapy in patients with nonrheumatic atrial fibrillation and recent cerebral ischemia. *N Engl J Med* 1995; 333:5–10

41. Vaitkus PT, Barnathan ES. Embolic potential, prevention and management of mural thrombus complicating anterior myocardial infarction: A meta-analysis. *J Am Coll Cardiol* 1993;22:1004–9

42. Jorgensen HS, Nakayama H, Raaschou HO, Larsen K, Hubbe P, Olsen TS. The effect of a stroke unit: Reductions in mortality, discharge rate to nursing home, length of hospital stay and cost. A community-based study. *Stroke* 1995;26:1178–82

43. Smith DS, Goldenberg E, Ashburn A, *et al.* Remedial therapy after stroke: A randomised controlled trial. *BMJ* 1981;282:517–20

44. Strand T, Apslund K, Eriksson S, Hagg E, Lithner F, Wester PO. A non-intensive stroke unit reduces functional disability and the need for long-term hospitalization. *Stroke* 1985;16:29–34

45. Ween JE, Alexander MP, D'Esposito M, Roberts M. Factors predictive of stroke outcome in a rehabilitation setting. *Neurology* 1996;47:388–92

46. Vinters HV. Cerebral amyloid angiopathy. A critical review. *Stroke* 1987;18:311–21

47. Furlan AJ, Kanoti G. When is thrombolysis justified in patients with acute ischemic stroke? *Stroke* 1997;28:214–8

48. Censori B, Manara O, Agostinis C, *et al.* Dementia after first stroke. Stroke 1996; 27:1205–10

49. Liao D, Couper L, Cai J, *et al.* Presence and severity of cerebral white matter lesions and hypertension, its treatment, and its control. The ARIC Study. *Stroke* 1996;27:2262–70

50. Longstreth WT, Manolio TA, Arnold A, *et al.,* for the Cardiovascular Health Study Collaborative Research Group. Clinical correlates of white matter findings on cranial magnetic resonance imaging of 3,301 elderly people: The Cardiovascular Health Study. *Stroke* 1996;27: 1274–82

51. Sacco RL, Benjamin EJ, Broderick JP, *et al.* Risk Factors Panel. American Heart Association Prevention Conference IV. *Stroke* 1997; 28:1507–17

52. Sacco RL, Boden-Albala B, Gan R, *et al.* and the Northern Manhattan Stroke Study Collaborators. Stroke incidence among white, black and Hispanic residents of an urban community: The Northern Manhattan Stroke Study. *Am J Epidemiol* 1998;147:259–68

53. Broderick J, Brott T, Kothari R, *et al.* The Greater Cincinnati/Northern Kentucky Stroke Study: Preliminary first-ever and total incidence rates of stroke among blacks. *Stroke* 1998;29: 415–21

54. Wolf PA, D'Agostino RB, Belanger AJ, Kannel WB. Probability of stroke: A risk profile from the Framingham Study. *Stroke* 1991;22: 312–8

55. MacMahon S, Rodgers A. The epidemiological association between blood pressure and stroke: Implications for primary and secondary prevention. *Hypertens Res* 1994;17(Suppl 1):S23–32

56. MacMahon S, Peto R, Cutler J, *et al.* Blood pressure, stroke, and coronary heart disease. Part 1: Prolonged differences in blood pressure: Prospective observational studies corrected for the regression dilution bias. *Lancet* 1990;335: 765–74

57. Collins R, Peto R, MacMahon S, *et al.* Blood pressure, stroke, and coronary heart disease. Part 2: Short-term reductions in blood pressure: Overview of randomised drug trials in their epidemiological context. *Lancet* 1990;335: 827–38

58. SHEP Cooperative Research Group. Prevention of stroke by antihypertensive drug treatment in older persons with isolated systolic hypertension: Final results of the Systolic Hypertension in the Elderly Program (SHEP). *JAMA* 1991; 265:3255–64

59. Staessen JA, Fagard R, Thijs L, *et al.* Randomised double-blind comparison of placebo and active treatment for older patients with isolated systolic hypertension. *Lancet* 1997;350:757–64

60. Tuomilehto J, Nissinen A, Wolf E, *et al.* Effectiveness of treatment with antihypertensive drugs and trends in mortality from stroke in the community. *Br Med J* 1985;291:857–61

61. Gorelick PB. Stroke prevention: Windows of opportunity and failed expectations – A discussion of modifiable cardiovascular risk factors and a prevention proposal. *Neuroepidemiology* 1997;16:163–73

62. Wolf PA, Abbott RD, Kannel WB. Atrial fibrillation as an independent risk factor for stroke: The Framingham Study. *Stroke* 1991;22:983–8

63. Atrial Fibrillation Investigators. Risk factors for stroke and efficacy of antithrombotic therapy in atrial fibrillation: Analysis of pooled data from five randomized controlled trials. *Arch Intern Med* 1994;154:1449–57

64. Stroke Prevention in Atrial Fibrillation Investigators. Adjusted-dose warfarin versus low-intensity, fixed-dose warfarin plus aspirin for high-risk patients with atrial fibrillation: Stroke Prevention in Atrial Fibrillation III randomised clinical trial. *Lancet* 1996;348:633–8

65. Laupacis A, Albers G, Dalen J, Dunn MI, Jacobson AK, Singer DE. Antithrombotic therapy in atrial fibrillation. *Chest* 1998;114:579–89S

66. Steering Committee of the Physicians' Health Study Research Group. Final report on the aspirin component of the ongoing Physicians' Health Study. *N Engl J Med* 1989;321:129–35

67. Peto R, Gray R, Collins R, *et al.* Randomised trial of prophylactic aspirin in British male doctors. *Br Med J* 1988;296:313–6

68. Barrett-Connor E, Khaw K.-T. Diabetes mellitus: An independent risk factor for stroke. *Am J Epidemiol* 1988;128:116–24

69. Tuomilehto J, Rastenyte MD, Jousilahti P, *et al.* Diabetes mellitus as a risk factor for death from stroke. *Stroke* 1996;27:210–5

70. The Diabetes Control and Complications Trial Research Group. The effect of intensive treatment of diabetes on the development and progression of long-term complications in insulin-dependent diabetes mellitus. *N Engl J Med* 1993;329:977–86

71. Prospective Studies Collaboration. Cholesterol, diastolic blood pressure, and stroke: 13,000 strokes in 450,000 people in 45 prospective cohorts. *Lancet* 1995;346:1647–53

72. Heiss G, Sharrett AR, Barnes R, *et al.* Carotid atherosclerosis measured by B-mode ultrasound in populations: Associations with cardiovascular risk factors in the ARIC study. *Am J Epidemiol* 1991;134:250–60

73. Hebert PR, Gaziano JM, Chan KS, Hennekens CH. Cholesterol lowering with statin drugs, risk of stroke, and total mortality: An overview of randomized trials. *JAMA* 1997;278:313–21

74. Shinton R, Beevers G. Meta-analysis of relation between cigarette smoking and stroke. *Br Med J* 1989;298:789–94

75. Kamachi I, Colditz GA, Stampfer MJ, *et al.* Smoking cessation and decreased risk of stroke in women. *JAMA* 1993;269:232–6

76. Sacco RL, Roberts JK, Boden-Albala B, *et al.* Race–ethnicity and determinants of carotid atherosclerosis in a multi-ethnic population: The Northern Manhattan Stroke Study. *Stroke* 1997;27:929–35

77. Camargo CA. Moderate alcohol consumption and stroke: The epidemiologic evidence. *Stroke* 1989;20:1611–26

78. Sacco R, Elkind M, Boden-Albala B, *et al.* The protective effect of moderate alcohol consumption on ischemic stroke. *JAMA* 1999;281:53–60

79. Abbott RD, Rodriguez BL, Burchfiel CM, Curb JD. Physical activity in older middle-aged men and reduced risk of stroke: The Honolulu Heart Program. *Am J Epidemiol* 1994;139:881–93

80. Kiely DK, Wolf PA, Cupples LA, *et al.* Physical activity and stroke risk: The Framingham Study. *Am J Epidemiol* 1994;140:608–20

81. Sacco RL, Gan R, Boden-Albala B, *et al.* Leisure-time physical activity and ischemic stroke risk: The Northern Manhattan Stroke Study. *Stroke* 1998;29:380–7

82. Pate RR, Pratt M, Blair SN, *et al.* Physical activity and public health: A recommendation from the Centers for Disease Control and Prevention and the American College of Sports Medicine. *JAMA* 1995;273:402–7

83. Chambers BR, Norris JW. Outcome in patients with asymptomatic neck bruits. *N Engl J Med* 1986;315:860–5

Further reading

Amar K, Wilcock G. Vascular dementia. *Br Med J* 1996;312:227–31

Bogousslavsky J, Caplan L, eds. *Stroke Syndromes.* Cambridge: Cambridge University Press, 1995

Bronner LL, Kanter DS, Manson JE. Primary prevention of stroke. *N Engl J Med* 1995;335:1392–1400

Brust JCM. Vascular dementia is overdiagnosed. *Arch Neurol* 1988;45:799–801

Jellinger K, Danielczyk W, Fischer P, Gabriel E. Clinicopathological analysis of dementia described in the elderly. *J Neurol Sci* 1990;95:239–58

Kase CS, Caplan LS, eds. *Intracerebral Haemorrhage.* Boston, London: Butterworth–Heinemann, 1994

Langhorne P, for Stroke Unit Trialists' Collaboration. Collaborative systematic review of the randomised trials of organised inpatient (stroke unit) care after stroke. *Br Med J* 1997;314:1151–9

O'Brien MD. Vascular dementia is underdiagnosed. *Arch Neurol* 1988;45:797–8

Stroke octet (series of papers)

Bamford J. Clinical examination in diagnosis and subclassification of stroke. *Lancet* 1992;339:400–5

Bonita R. Epidemiology of stroke. *Lancet* 1992; 339:342–4

Caplan LR. Intracerebral haemorrhage. *Lancet* 1992; 339:656–8

Donnan GA. Investigation of patients with stroke and transient ischaemic attacks. *Lancet* 1992;339: 473–7

van Gijn J. Subarachnoid haemorrhage. *Lancet* 1992; 339:653–5

Hart RG. Cardiogenic embolism to the brain. *Lancet* 1992;339:489–594

Landi G. Clinical diagnosis of transient ischaemic attacks. *Lancet* 1992;339:402–5

Marmot MG, Poulter NR. Primary prevention of stroke. *Lancet* 1992;339:344–7

Oppenheimer S, Hachinski V. Complications of acute stroke. *Lancet* 1992;339:721–4

Pulsinelli W. Pathophysiology of acute ischaemic stroke. *Lancet* 1992;339:533–6

Sandercock P, Willems H. Medical treatment of acute ischaemic stroke. *Lancet* 1992;339:537–9

Section 2   Stroke Illustrated

List of illustrations

Classification of stroke (1)

Oxford

Anterior circulation
Total (TACI)
Partial (PACI)

Posterior circulation (POCI)

Lacunar (LACI)

Stroke Data Bank

Large artery atherosclerosis

Lacunar

Cardioembolic

Tandem arterial lesions

Unknown etiology

Other

Figure 1 Two schemes for the classification of ischemic strokes

Classification of stroke (2)

National Institute of Neurological Diseases and Stroke

Clinical
Atherothrombotic
Cardioembolic
Lacunar
Arterial territory
Internal carotid
Middle cerebral
Anterior cerebral
Vertebral
Basilar
Posterior cerebral
Mechanism
Thrombotic
Embolic
Hemodynamic

Figure 2 Another scheme for the classification of ischemic strokes

Causes of acute ischemic stroke and transient ischemic attacks

Atherothrombosis

Disease of small medullary arteries
Hypertension
Diabetes mellitus
CADASIL syndrome: Familial syndrome with autosomal-dominant inheritance leading to early subcortical stroke and vascular dementia

Necrotizing arteritis (including Takayasu's disease)

Arterial dissection (trauma, but may be familial)

Cardiac embolism due to
Acute myocardial infarction (especially anterior)
Left ventricular aneurysm, dyskinetic segment
Poor function
Atrial dilatation / fibrillation
Infective endocarditis
Non-infective endocarditis
Atrial myxoma

Artery-to-artery embolism due to
Atherosclerosis of aorta or of large arteries, including arterial dissection

Paradoxical embolism

Hypercoagulable states
Thrombocytosis and myeloproliferative diseases
Thrombophilias (much more likely to develop cerebral venous thrombosis)
Factor V Leiden
Deficiency of protein C or S
Lupus anticoagulant
Antiphospholipid antibodies

Vasospasm
Drug-induced
Delayed after subarachnoid hemorrhage

Acute and chronic infections

Migraine-associated

Figure 3 Vascular causes of ischemic stroke

Risk factors for ischemic stroke

Non-modifiable risk markers
Older age
Male gender
Race and ethnicity
Genetic factors

Modifiable risk factors
Hypertension
Diabetes mellitus
Hyperlipidemia
Cigarette-smoking
Excessive alcohol consumption
Physical inactivity
Carotid artery stenosis
Cardiac conditions
Atrial fibrillation
Myocardial infarction
Left ventricular dysfunction
Valvular heart disease
Left ventricular hypertrophy

Potential risk factors
Antiphospholipid antibodies
Homocysteine
Infection
Systemic inflammation
Migraine
Oral contraceptive use
Sympathomimetics
Illicit drug use
Obesity
Diet (fat, antioxidants, supplemental vitamins)
Stress
Ankle-to-brachial blood pressure ratio
MRI white matter abnormalities
Cardiac conditions
Patent foramen ovale
Atrial septal aneurysm
Mitral annular calcification
Mitral valve strands
Aortic arch atheroma

Therapeutic recommendations for ischemic stroke subtypes

Subtype	Therapy
Atherosclerotic carotid disease	
• ≥ 70% stenosis	Carotid endarterectomy (CEA) of proven efficacy as long as operative risk is low
	Follow-up CEA with antiplatelet therapy*
	Angioplasty with stent in clinical trials as alternative to CEA
• 50–69% stenosis	Antiplatelet therapy*
	Consider CEA depending on patient's risk factor profile
• < 50% stenosis	Antiplatelet therapy*
	CEA not indicated
Cardiac embolism	
• Known source, such as:	Oral anticoagulant (except when contraindicated):
Left ventricular thrombus, recent myocardial infarction	6 months of therapy, INR 2–3 with a target of 2.5
Non-valvular atrial fibrillation	Life-long therapy, INR 2–3 with a target of 2.5
Prosthetic valvular heart disease	Life-long therapy, INR 3–4 with a target of 3.5
• Unknown or indefinite source	Antiplatelet therapy*; oral anticoagulants in clinical trials as alternative therapy
Other infarct subtypes such as small-vessel lacunar disease and cryptogenic stroke	Antiplatelet therapy*; oral anticoagulants in clinical trials as alternative therapy

> *Antiplatelet agents (listed alphabetically)
> Aspirin; Clopidogrel (Plavix®);
> Extended-release dipyridamole plus aspirin (Aggrenox®); Ticlopidine (Ticlid®)

Figure 4 Risk factors for ischemic stroke and therapeutic recommendations for ischemic stroke subtypes

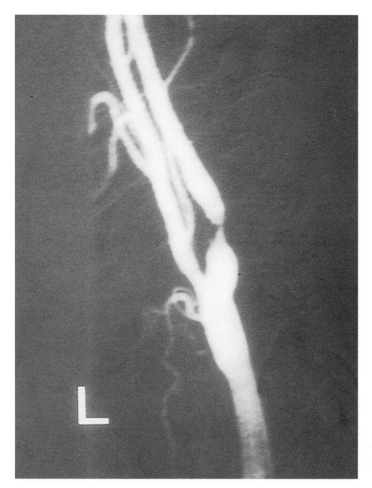

Figure 5 Angiogram showing a severe stenosis in the left internal carotid artery. The patient presented with a transient right hemiparesis

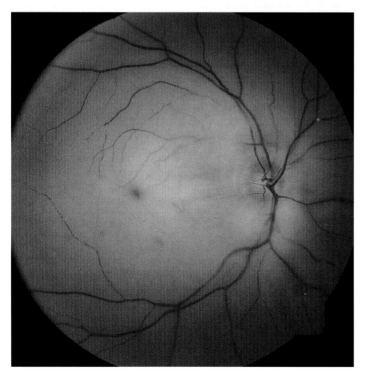

Figure 6 Funduscopy showing a central retinal artery occlusion, a condition that is usually due to atheroembolism. The evidence for an artery-to-artery embolism in this retina is the refractile so-called Hollenhorst plaque lodged at a point of arterial bifurcation in the nasal retina (arrowed). Amaurosis fugax is commonly the result of embolism from an internal carotid artery stenosis

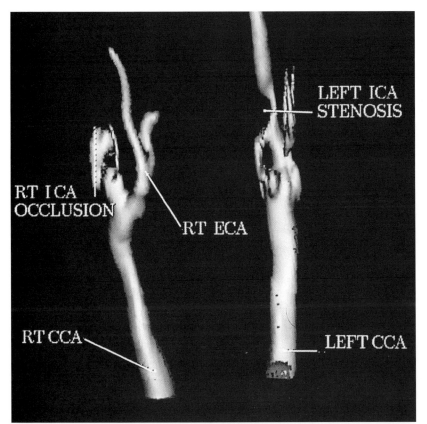

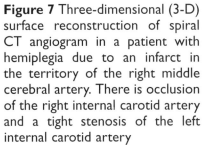

Figure 7 Three-dimensional (3-D) surface reconstruction of spiral CT angiogram in a patient with hemiplegia due to an infarct in the territory of the right middle cerebral artery. There is occlusion of the right internal carotid artery and a tight stenosis of the left internal carotid artery

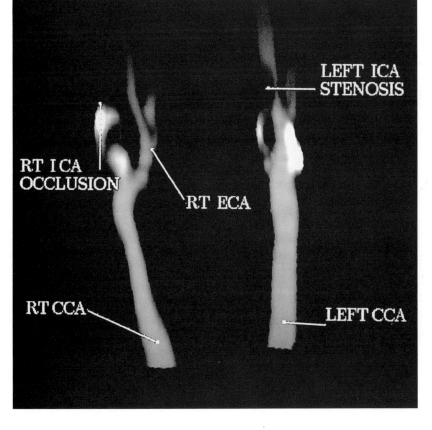

Figure 8 Maximum-intensity projection of the same scan as in Figure 7 clearly shows both lesions as well as areas of vascular calcification

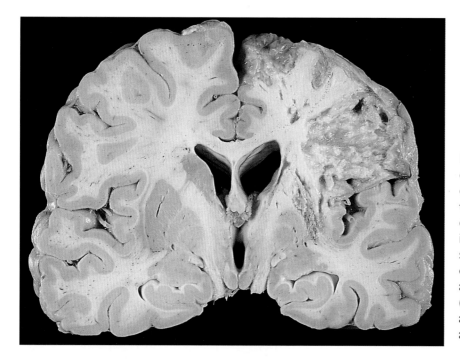

Figure 9 Coronal section of cerebral cortex showing softening due to infarction in the territory of the left middle cerebral artery. The putamen is clearly involved. The corresponding clinical syndrome is often referred to as a total anterior circulation infarct (TACI), and is associated with a poor prognosis for survival and functional outcome

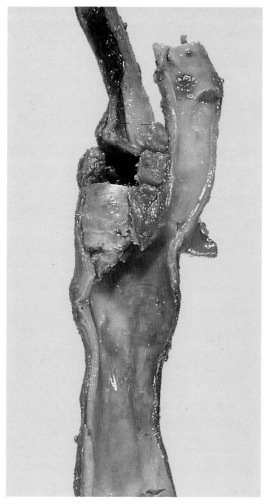

Figure 10 This internal carotid artery is occluded with thrombus superimposed on an atherosclerotic plaque. Approximately 30% of infarcts in the middle cerebral artery territory are caused by extracranial arterial disease. Depending on the adequacy of collateral flow and especially on the size of the posterior communicating artery, the extent of infarction after carotid occlusion varies considerably

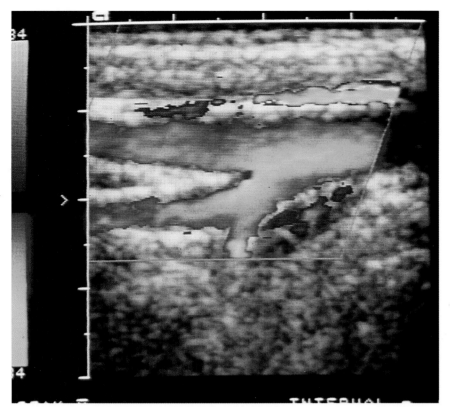

Figure 11 Color Doppler imaging (CDI) of a normal carotid bifurcation. The common carotid artery (on the right) is clearly seen dividing into the internal (lower left) and external (upper left) carotid arteries. Normal flow velocity appears blue

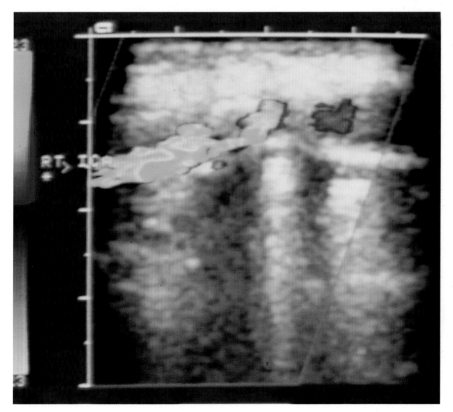

Figure 12 CDI of a stenosis at the origin of the internal carotid artery. The common carotid artery (on the right) has a normal velocity of flow indicated by red. Increased velocities of flow through and distal to the stenosis are visualized as yellow and green

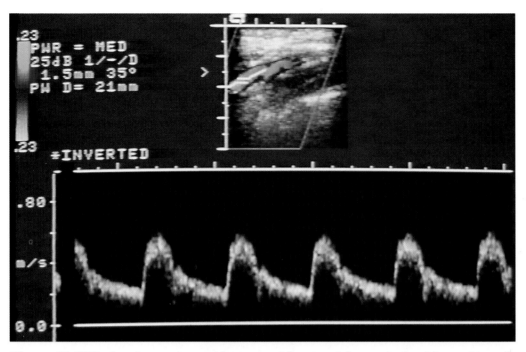

Figure 13 CDI of an internal carotid artery with normal flow velocity (shown by red). The Doppler signatures in the artery through several cardiac cycles are displayed below. The pulsed Doppler frequency spectrum shows a narrow range of frequencies with rounded peaks during systole and an average velocity 0.6 m / s (normal < 1.0)

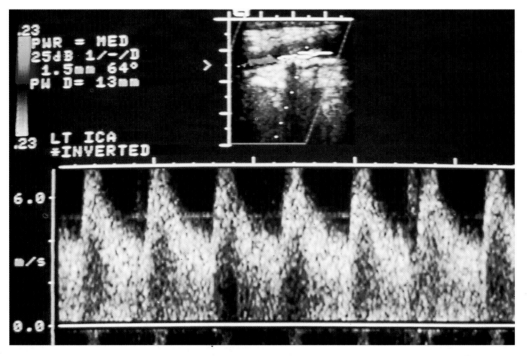

Figure 14 CDI showing Doppler signatures of a severely stenosed internal carotid artery. There is a marked increase in peak velocity to > 6 m / s (normal < 1.0) and a sharp peak. Flow disturbance is also indicated by the much wider range of velocities reflected by the broadening of the spectrum compared with normal

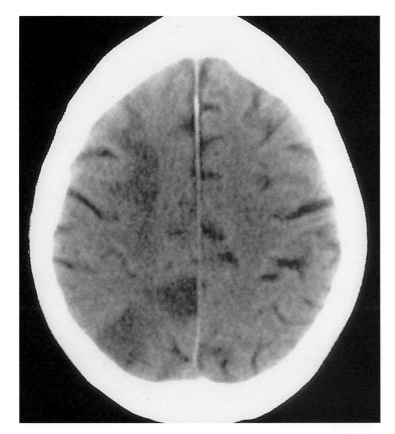

Figure 15 CT showing border-zone or 'watershed' cortical infarcts in a patient with occlusion of the right internal carotid artery. The border zones between the territories of the middle and anterior cerebral arteries, and middle and posterior cerebral arteries, respectively, are vulnerable when carotid pressure is greatly reduced. As there is considerable variation among individuals in respective arterial territories, border-zone infarcts are not always as easy to recognize

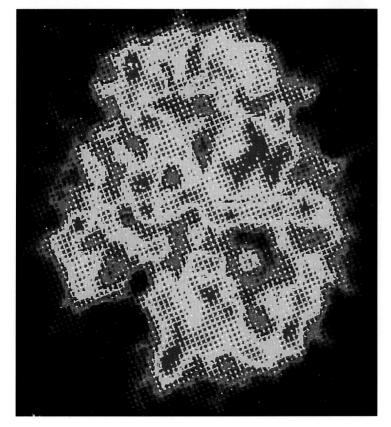

Figure 16 Technetium 99m-hexamethyl-propylene amine oxide (HMPAO) and single-photon emission tomography (SPECT) (same patient as in Figure 15) showing the area of reduced perfusion associated with the more posterior infarct. More anteriorly, a smaller area of reduced perfusion is just discernible

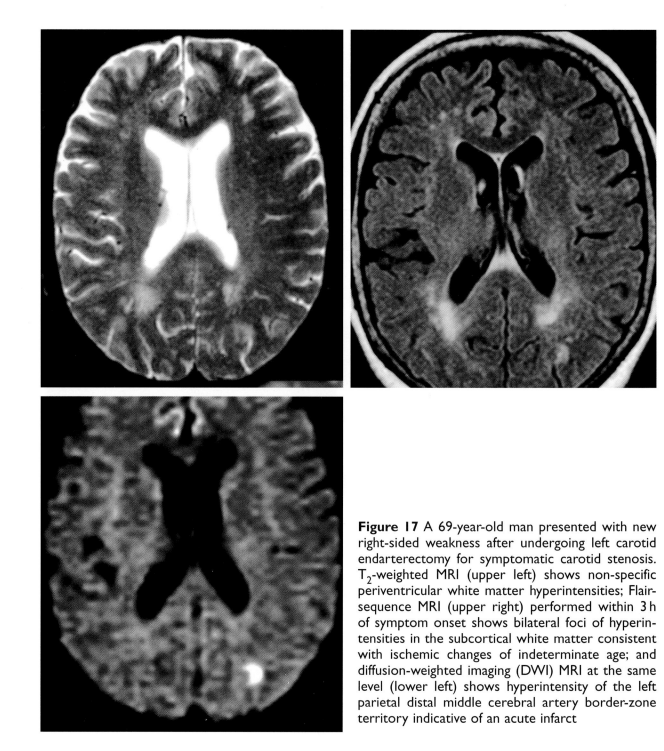

Figure 17 A 69-year-old man presented with new right-sided weakness after undergoing left carotid endarterectomy for symptomatic carotid stenosis. T_2-weighted MRI (upper left) shows non-specific periventricular white matter hyperintensities; Flair-sequence MRI (upper right) performed within 3 h of symptom onset shows bilateral foci of hyperintensities in the subcortical white matter consistent with ischemic changes of indeterminate age; and diffusion-weighted imaging (DWI) MRI at the same level (lower left) shows hyperintensity of the left parietal distal middle cerebral artery border-zone territory indicative of an acute infarct

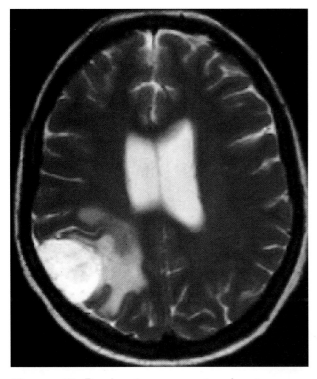

Figure 18 Focal seizures causing hemi-sensory symptoms may be mistaken for transient ischemic attacks (TIAs). This parietal meningioma, shown here on T$_2$-weighted MRI, resulted in left-sided symptoms which were misdiagnosed as TIAs

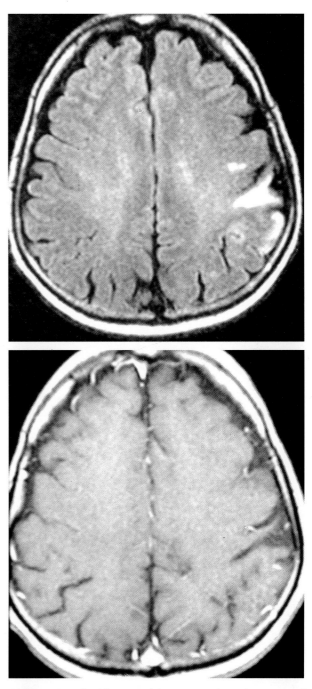

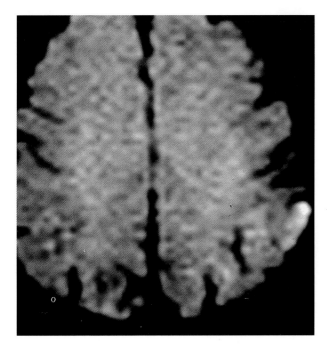

Figure 19 A 62-year-old man with a history of cancer presented with new weakness in his right hand. Flair-sequence MRI (upper) shows hyperintensity in the left parietal region which could represent an acute infarct or tumor edema. Contrast-enhanced T$_1$-weighted MRI (lower) failed to show signs of metastasis. DWI MRI (left) shows hyperintensity in the left parietal region that is consistent with cytotoxic edema due to an acute infarct and not tumor edema

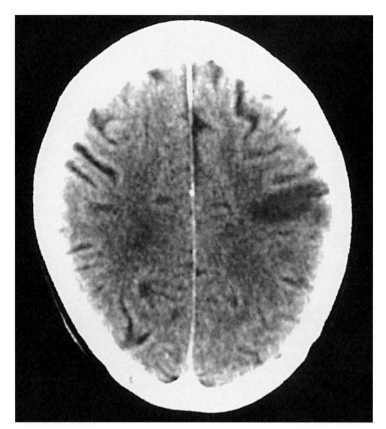

Figure 20 CT showing infarction in the territory of the central branch of the left middle cerebral artery which presented as mild weakness and numbness of the right arm. The infarct was probably caused by artery-to-artery embolism from a proximal internal carotid stenosis

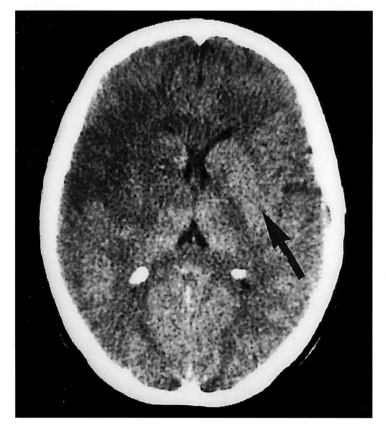

Figure 21 Early changes of infarction are difficult to detect on CT. In this 34-year-old patient, increased attenuation can be seen in the right middle cerebral artery territory due to increased water content of ischemic tissue. There is loss of definition of the corresponding lentiform nucleus (normal nucleus is arrowed)

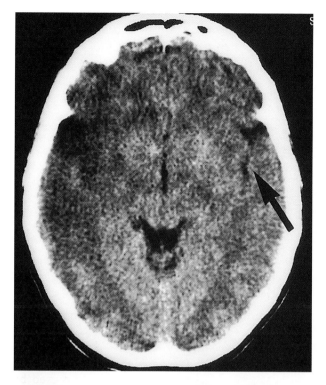

Figure 22 On CT, another useful sign of infarction can be seen here in the territory of the middle cerebral artery – loss of the ribbon deep in the Sylvian fissure (normal ribbon is arrowed)

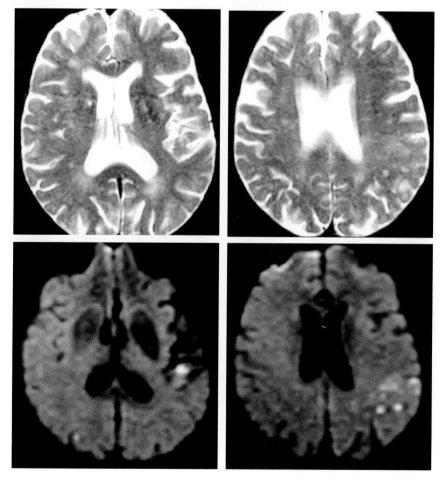

Figure 23 A 77-year-old woman presented with new speech disturbance which was clinically difficult to distinguish as dysarthria or aphasia. T_2-weighted MRIs taken at two levels (upper left and right) show non-specific white matter hyperintensities; however, DWI MRIs taken at the same levels (lower left and right) clearly reveal several left posterior Sylvian hyperintensities consistent with acute cortical infarction

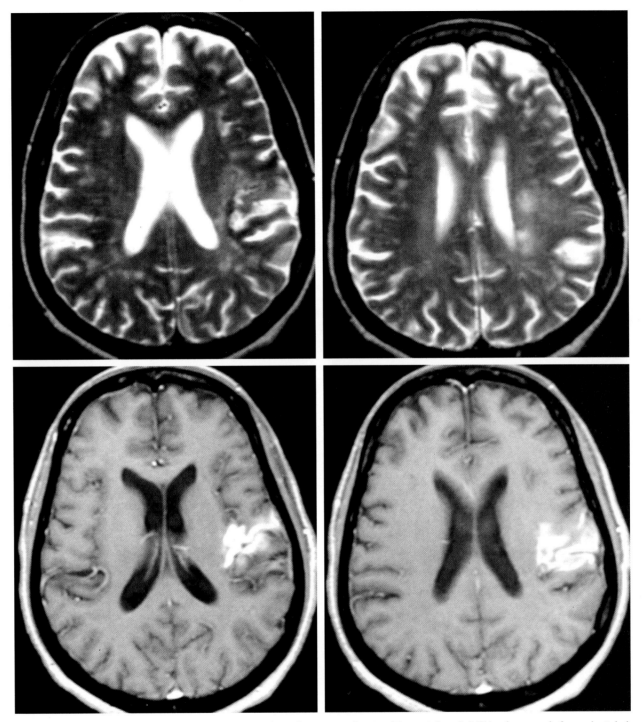

Figure 24 A 54-year-old woman presented with new aphasia. T_2-weighted MRIs (upper left and right) show abnormal signal intensities in the posterior left opercular region with minimal edema. Gadolinium-enhanced T_1-weighted MRIs (lower left and right) clearly demonstrate gyriform enhancement consistent with sub-acute infarction

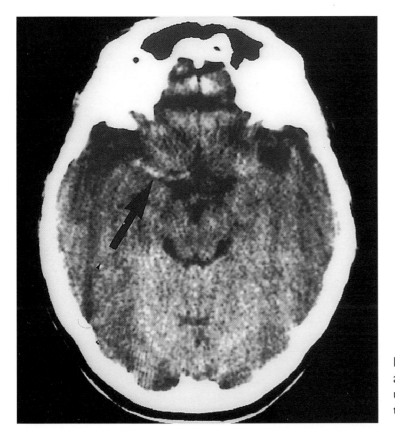

Figure 25 CT showing middle cerebral artery occlusion. There is increased attenuation in the stem of the artery, referred to as the 'string sign'

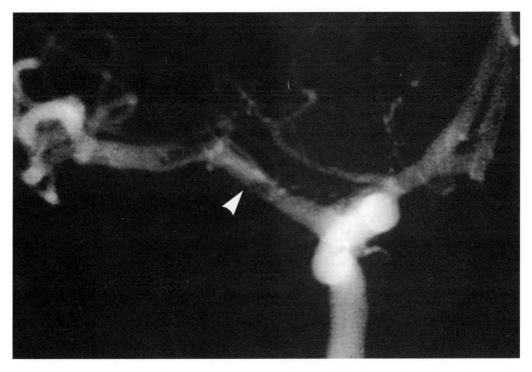

Figure 26 Angiography (same patient as in Figure 25) shows thrombus (arrowed) causing partial occlusion of the proximal middle cerebral artery

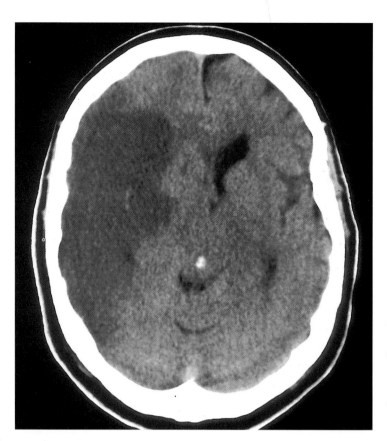

Figure 27 CT of a patient who experienced a progressive loss of consciousness 3 days after onset of right middle cerebral artery infarction. This was due to raised intracranial pressure as a result of edema around the infarct, visualized here as effacement of the ventricles and a midline shift. The term 'malignant middle cerebral artery syndrome' is sometimes used to describe this serious complication

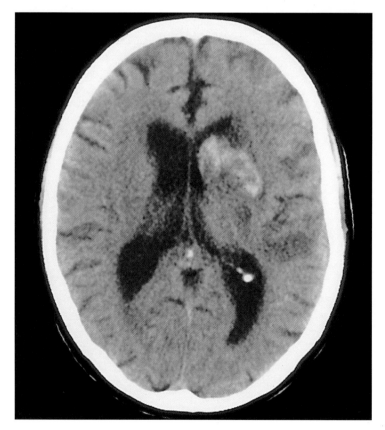

Figure 28 CT showing an infarct that is both deep and superficial in the left middle cerebral artery territory, and which has undergone hemorrhagic transformation in the region of the caudate nucleus. The scan was prompted by clinical deterioration 3 days after the onset of hemiplegia. Larger infarcts are more susceptible to hemorrhage

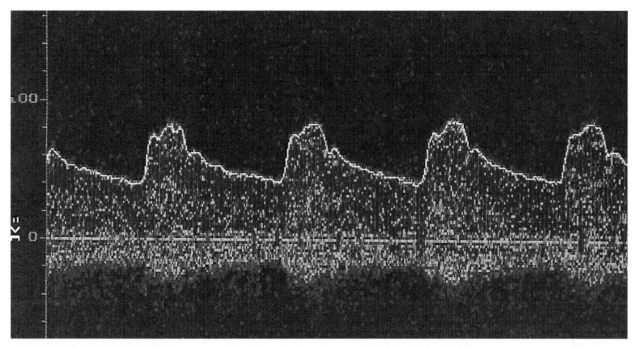

Figure 29 Transcranial CDI signature demonstrating a normal spectrum of velocities in the middle cerebral artery

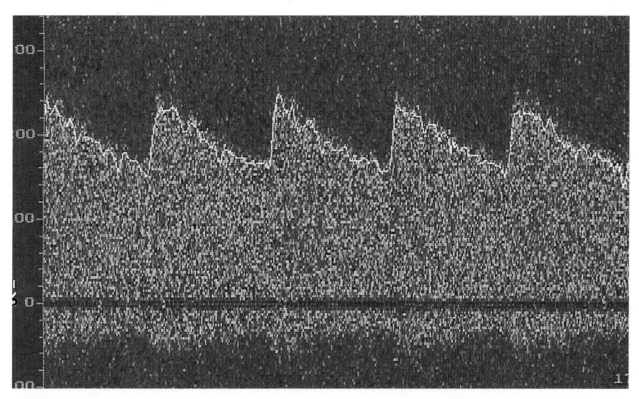

Figure 30 Transcranial CDI signature of a middle cerebral artery shows a highly abnormal pattern with much increased velocities as a result of partial occlusion

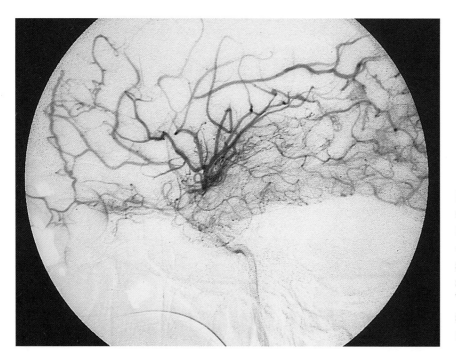

Figure 31 Carotid angiogram of an 18-year-old girl who had recurrent cerebral ischemic events showing neovascularization at the base of the brain and extending posteriorly. The 'puff of smoke' appearance is diagnostic of moyamoya syndrome

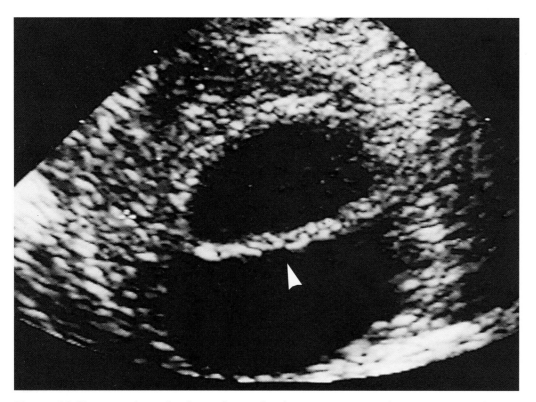

Figure 32 Transesophageal echocardiography showing an aortic dissection extending to the distal arch. The intimal flap is clearly seen (arrowed), and there is thrombus in the false lumen to the left and above. Aortic dissection is an uncommon cause of cerebral infarction and an occasional cause of spinal cord infarction

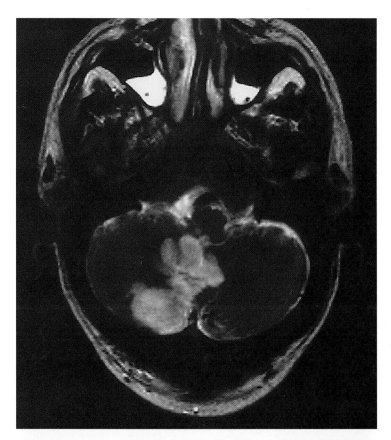

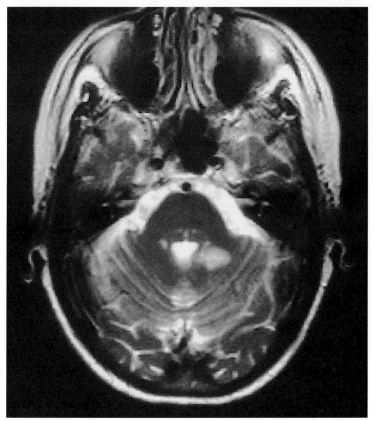

Figure 33 T$_1$-weighted MRI showing infarction of the cerebellum and lateral medulla in the territory supplied by the posterior inferior cerebellar artery and causing Wallenberg's syndrome. Occlusion in such cases is usually proximal in the vertebral artery and may be due to either atherosclerosis or cardioembolism. Dissection of the vertebral artery in the neck, sometimes caused by trauma, is a relatively rare but well-recognized cause

Figure 34 T$_2$-weighted MRI showing infarction confined to the lateral medulla, the result of vertebral artery occlusion

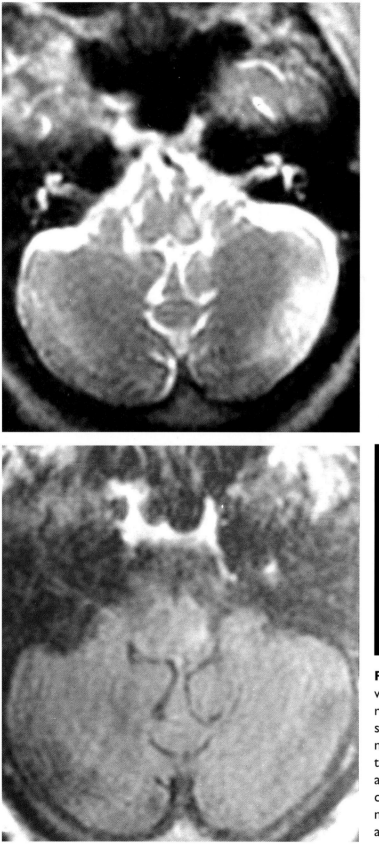

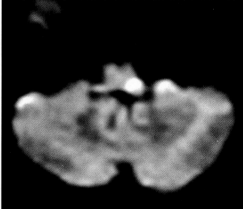

Figure 35 A 75-year-old man presented with a left Wallenberg's syndrome. High-resolution T$_2$-weighted MRI (upper left) shows a faint abnormality in the left lateral medulla. Flair-sequence MRI (lower left) at the same level also fails to show a clear abnormality, but DWI MRI (above) more convincingly demonstrates the left lateral medullary hyperintensity consistent with acute infarction

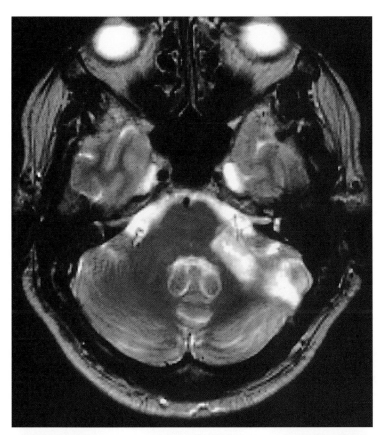

Figure 36 T$_2$-weighted MRI showing infarction of the cerebellum in the territory of the anterior inferior cerebellar artery. This sometimes leads to a clinical syndrome which is characterized by ipsilateral incoordination, tinnitus, dysarthria, facial weakness, hearing loss, loss of sensation in the trigeminal area, Horner's syndrome and contralateral loss of spinothalamic sensation

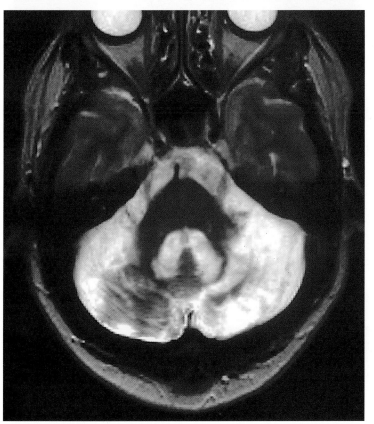

Figure 37 T$_2$-weighted MRI showing bilateral infarction of the cerebellum due to cardioembolism. Infarction that is confined to the superior cerebellar artery is usually a result of embolism

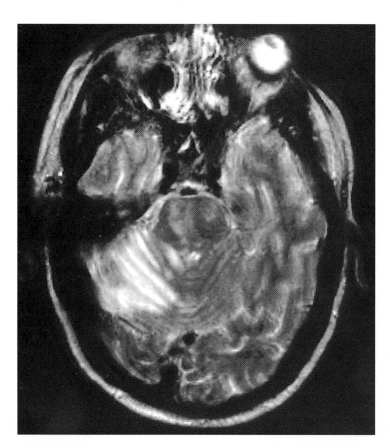

Figure 38 T$_1$-weighted MRI of a 52-year-old hypertensive cigarette smoker who has developed brain-stem infarction due to basilar artery occlusion. There is extensive infarction of the pons and right superior cerebellum. By this stage of disease, the patient showed quadriplegia and skew deviation of the eyes

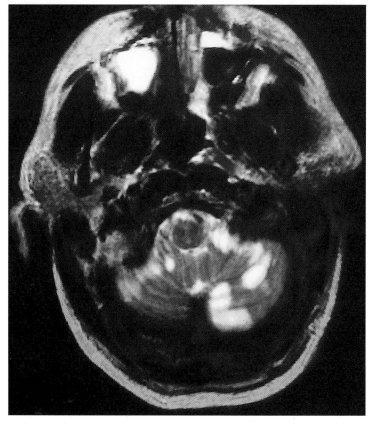

Figure 39 T$_1$-weighted MRI (same patient as in Figure 38) at a lower level shows widespread patchy cerebellar infarction

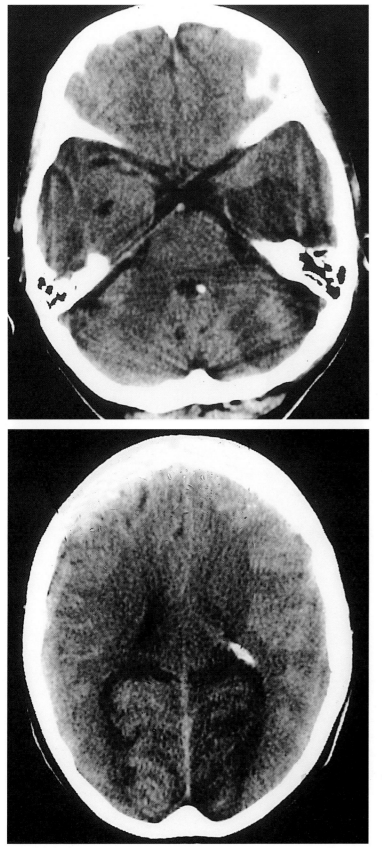

Figure 40 CTs showing infarction due to embolic occlusion of the basilar artery which is particularly marked in both cerebellar hemispheres as well as in the lower part of the left temporal lobe (upper) and in the occipital cortex (lower)

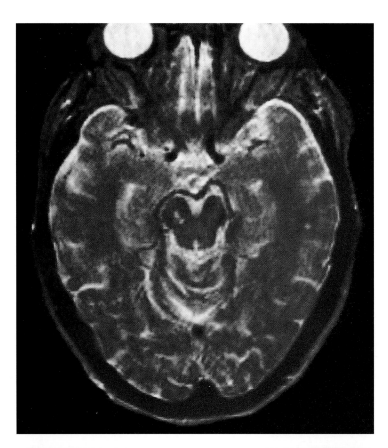

Figure 41 T$_2$-weighted MRI of a hypertensive patient who developed a small midbrain infarct. The clinical features included a right oculomotor palsy and contralateral incoordination (Claude's syndrome)

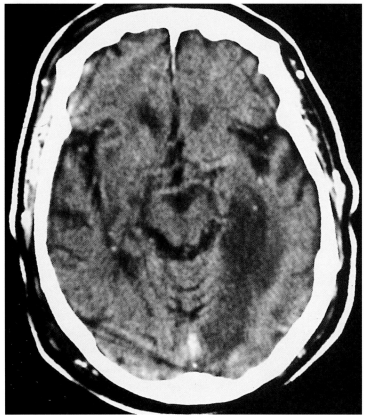

Figure 42 CT showing atherothrombotic occlusion of the posterior cerebral artery which has resulted in an infarction of the occipital cortex extending to the temporal lobe. Clinical features included agitation, persistent amnesia and a Wernicke's aphasia of transcortical type

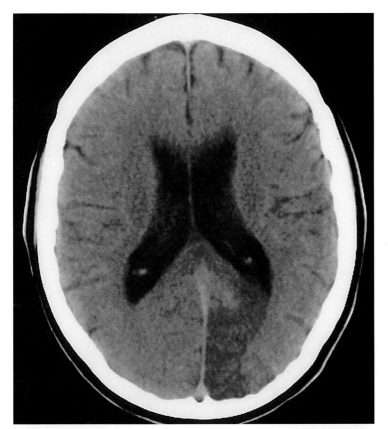

Figure 43 CT showing infarction of the left occipital cortex with resultant hemianopia in a 58-year-old patient with thrombophlebitis migrans subsequently shown to be associated with metastatic carcinoma of the pancreas

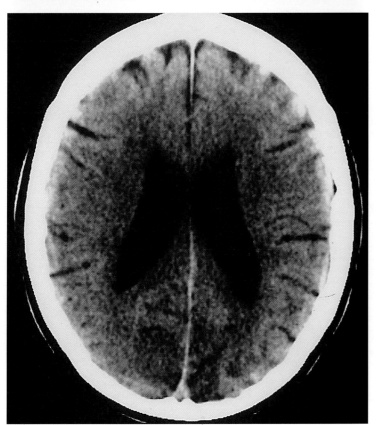

Figure 44 CT (same patient as in Figure 43) showing the later development of an infarction of the contralateral occipital cortex which left the patient with only central vision. It is likely that a coagulopathy was responsible, although cardioembolism was also considered

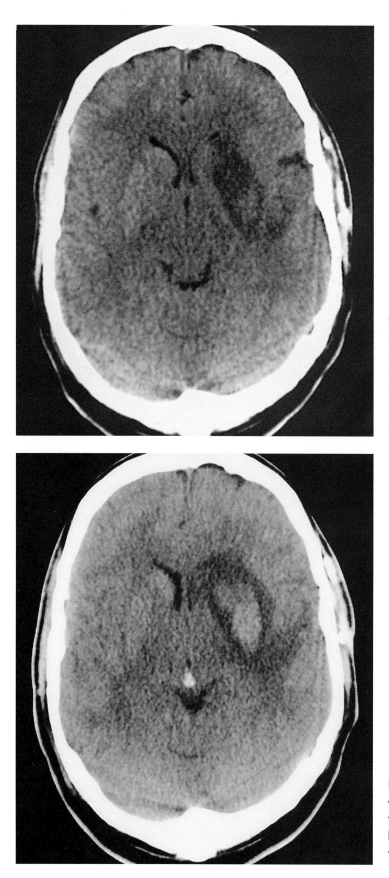

Figure 45 CT of a 33-year-old patient who presented with sudden-onset severe motor hemiplegia. The infarction is predominantly striatocapsular, characteristic of occlusion of the proximal middle cerebral artery and usually the result of embolism. Within the infarct, there is a small area of hemorrhagic transformation

Figure 46 CT (same patient as in Figure 45) taken on the following day shows that the hemorrhagic transformation has become more extensive, presumably due to reperfusion

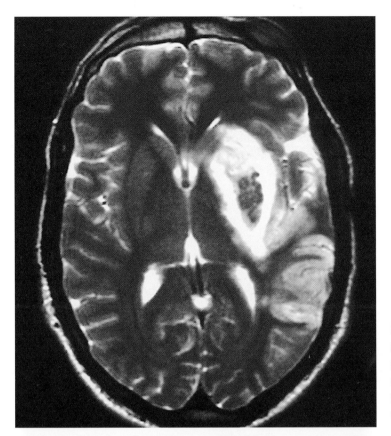

Figure 47 T$_2$-weighted MRI (same patient as in Figure 45) taken 4 days after onset shows hemorrhage surrounded by edema or infarction. There is also evidence of ischemia in the peripheral territories of the middle cerebral artery

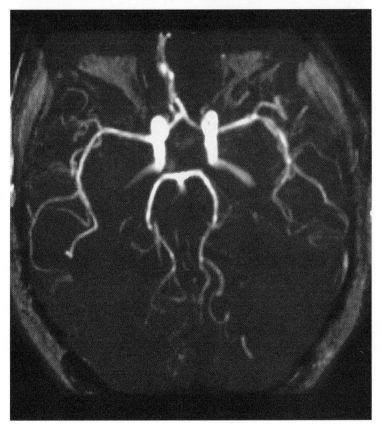

Figure 48 MRI angiography (same patient as in Figure 45) taken at the same stage of disease shows that middle cerebral artery patency has been restored

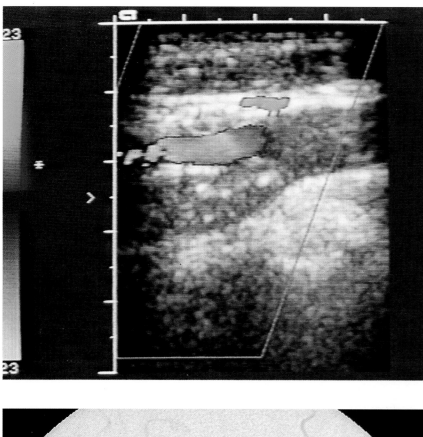

Figure 49 CDI shows normal flow in the external carotid artery (orange) whereas the internal carotid artery (below and to the left) is occluded by thrombus which, in this case, was due to embolism from an acute anterior myocardial infarction

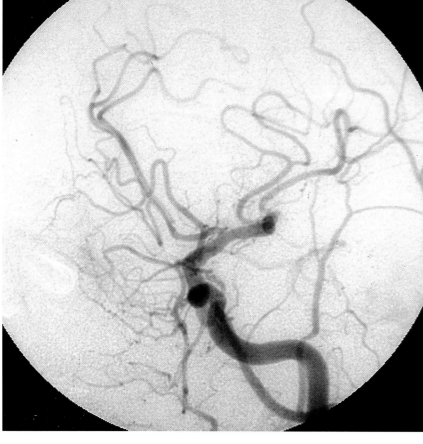

Figure 50 Angiogram of the left carotid artery showing an absence of flow in the lower division of the middle cerebral artery due to cardiogenic embolism. Strokes of this type usually result in Wernicke's aphasia and are most often due to cardiogenic or artery-to-artery embolism

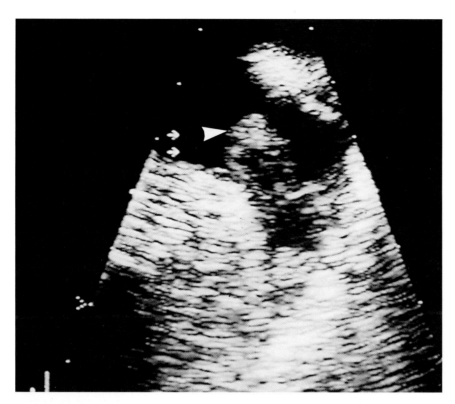

Figure 51 Transesophageal echocardiography of an 80-year-old patient who had atrial flutter/fibrillation and multiple cerebral infarcts on CT. A mobile thrombus (arrowed) can be seen in the left atrial appendage

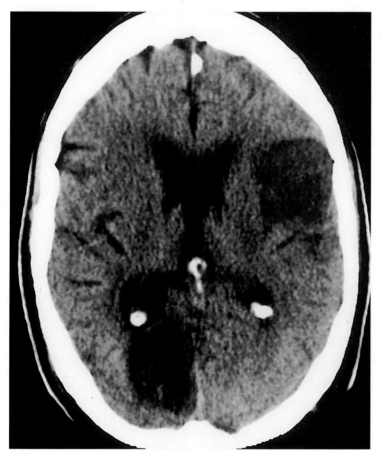

Figure 52 CT (same patient as in Figure 51) showing cerebral cortical infarcts. The infarct in the occipital lobe is old whereas that in the superficial middle cerebral territory is relatively recent. Both were caused by embolism

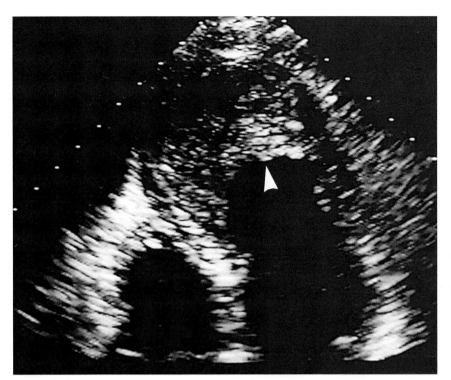

Figure 53 Transthoracic echo-cardiography of a 50-year-old patient 3 weeks after Q-wave anterior myocardial infarction reveals a mass of thrombus (arrowed) in an aneurysmal dilatation at the apex of the left ventricle

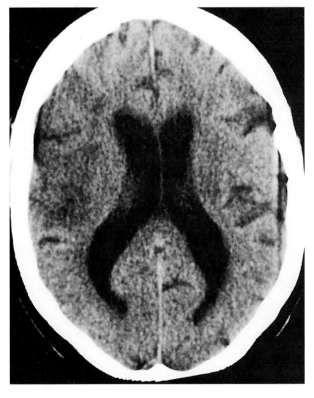

Figure 54 CT (same patient as in Figure 53) showing early changes of infarction in the right middle cerebral artery territory after sudden onset of left hemiplegia, hemisensory loss and hemianopia

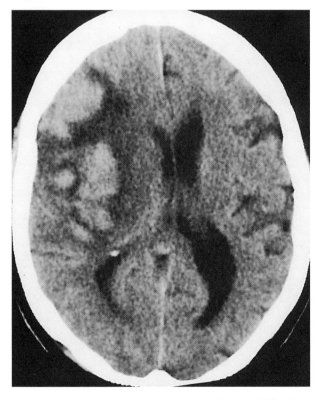

Figure 55 CT (same patient as in Figure 53) after clinical deterioration 48 h later shows extensive hemorrhagic transformation. Infarcts resulting from embolism are prone to such transformation

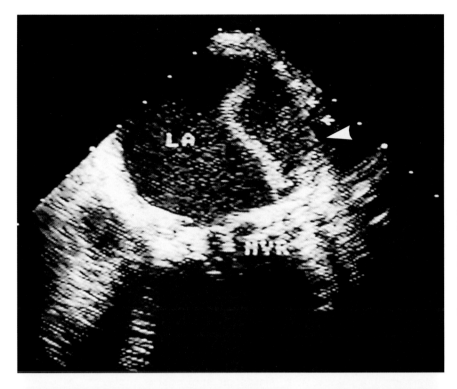

Figure 56 Transesophageal echocardiography of a 57-year-old patient with atrial fibrillation who developed a severe posterior circulation stroke due to cardiogenic embolism. There is thrombus (arrowed) in the left atrium and adjacent 'spontaneous contrast', an appearance that is probably the result of stagnant blood flow

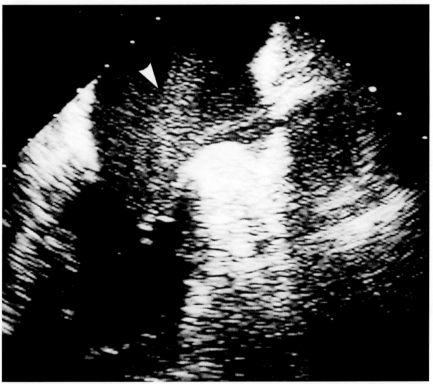

Figure 57 Transesophageal echocardiography showing the appearance of 'spontaneous contrast' (arrowed) in the left atrium of a patient with atrial fibrillation and suspected embolic stroke

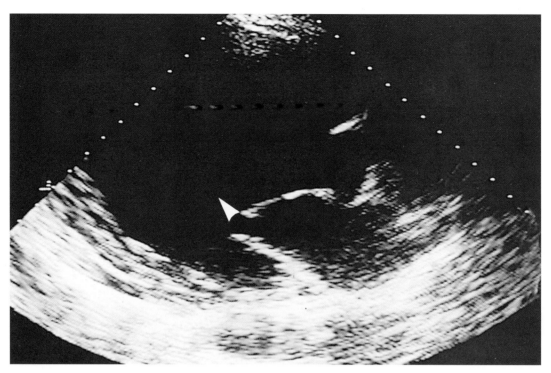

Figure 58 Transthoracic echocardiography in a patient with dilated cardiomyopathy shows a greatly enlarged left ventricle (arrowed) which was contracting very poorly. The risk of embolic stroke in this type of patient is high

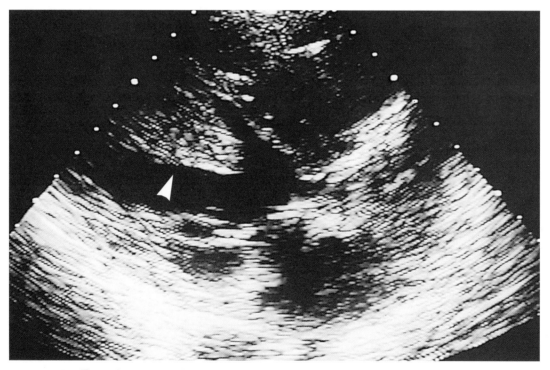

Figure 59 Transthoracic echocardiography of a patient following anterior myocardial infarction demonstrates a thrombus (arrowed) in the left ventricle. Anterior myocardial infarction carries a much higher risk of embolism compared with inferior infarction

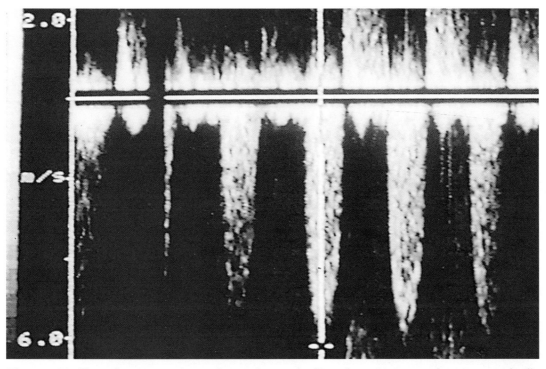

Figure 60 Transthoracic echocardiography with Doppler signature showing markedly increased aortic systolic flow, reaching nearly 6 m/s, due to severe aortic stenosis. Calcific aortic stenosis and mitral annulus calcification have been suspected to cause embolic stroke

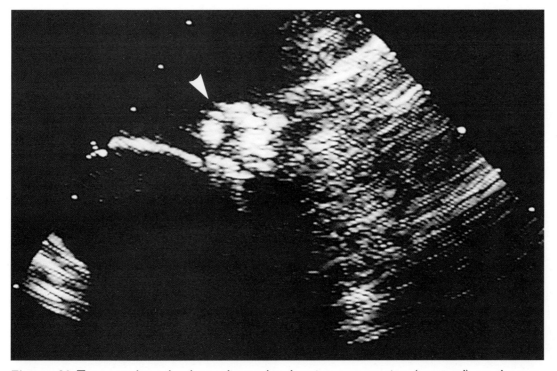

Figure 61 Transesophageal echocardiography showing a vegetation (arrowed) on the posterior leaflet of the mitral valve. Vegetations due to infective endocarditis may cause embolic stroke

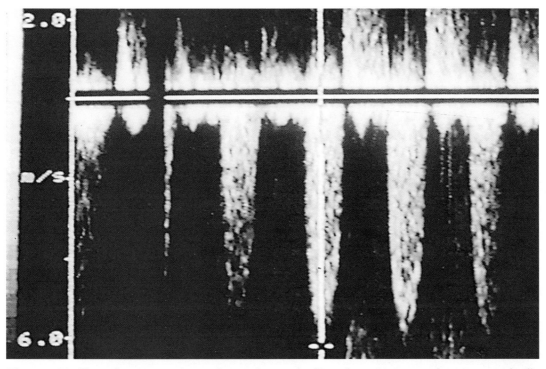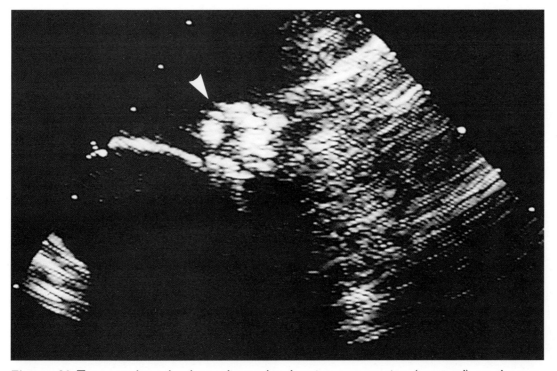

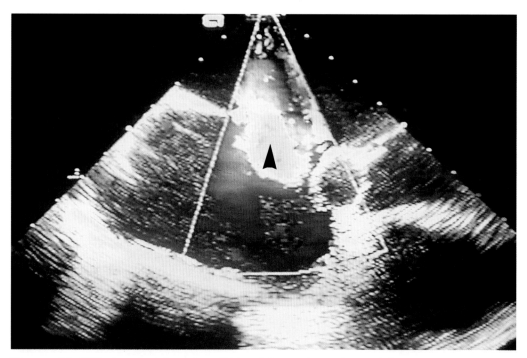

Figure 62 CDI showing shunting of blood from the right to left atrium *via* a patent foramen ovale (arrowed). The increased velocity of blood flow is indicated by yellow. Patients with shunts are at risk of paradoxical embolism. Another technique to demonstrate this type of shunt uses transcranial Doppler monitoring after intravenous injection of microbubbles

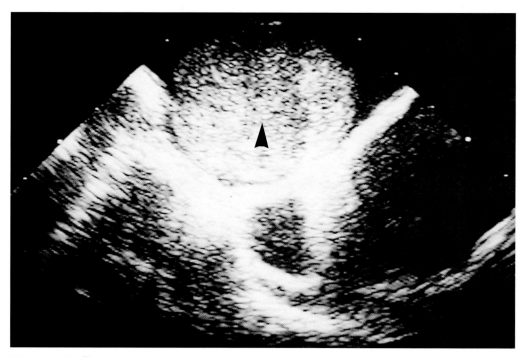

Figure 63 Transesophageal echocardiography showing a large left atrial myxoma (arrowed) in a patient who presented with transient cerebral ischemic attacks presumably due to emboli from the tumor

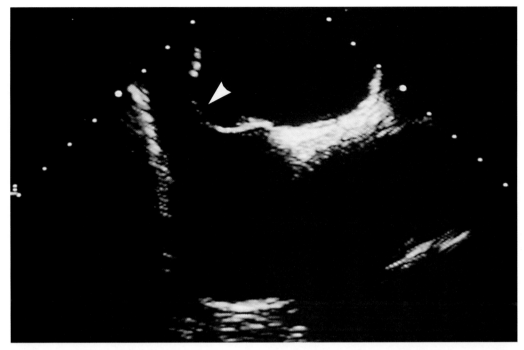

Figure 64 Transesophageal echocardiography showing an aneurysmal area in the interatrial septum (arrowed), seen bulging towards the right atrium, of a patient who presented with transient ischemic attacks. Abnormalities in this area may predispose to embolism

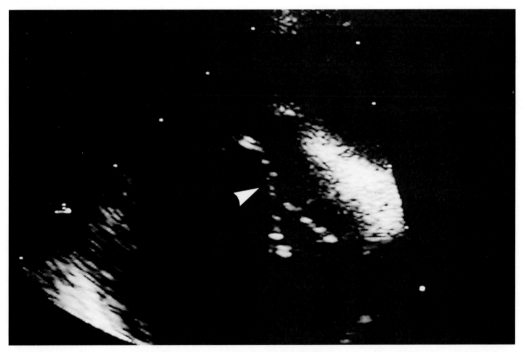

Figure 65 Transesophageal echocardiography showing a filamentous structure or Chiari network (arrowed) in the left atrium. Such an appearance has been suspected to predispose to embolism

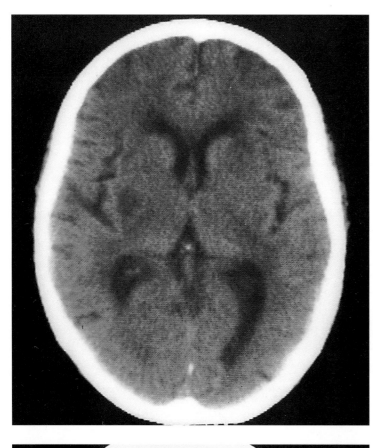

Figure 66 CT showing a small area of increased attenuation in the right basal ganglia due to a small deeply lying infarct, resulting from occlusion of a single penetrating artery. The pathological term lacune is used to describe a slit-like space in deep-lying white matter caused by single penetrating artery occlusion, small hemorrhages or a dilated perivascular space

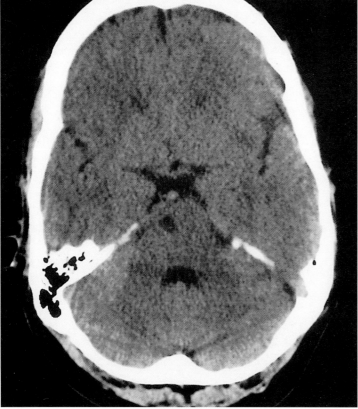

Figure 67 CT showing a lacunar infarct of the right basis pontis in a 41-year-old patient presenting with ataxic hemiparesis on the left side. The patient had severe hypertension

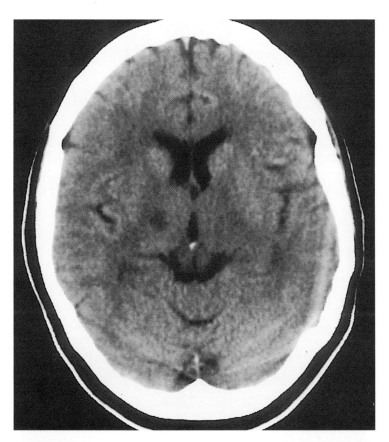

Figure 68 CT showing a lacunar infarct of the right lateral thalamus in a 51-year-old patient with severe hypertension who presented with pure sensory stroke. The infarct has probably resulted from an occlusion of a perforator from the thalamogeniculate artery originating from the posterior cerebral artery

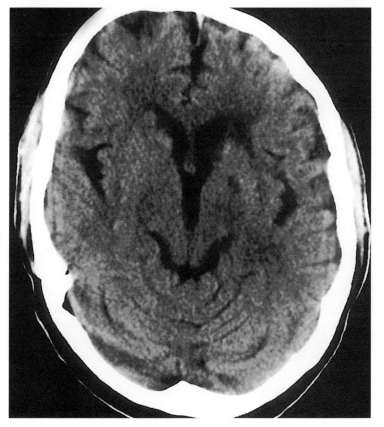

Figure 69 CT showing a very small deep infarct in the left internal capsule in a 63-year-old patient with hypertension and a transient (<24 h) pure motor weakness affecting the contralateral face, arm and leg. Many such lacunar infarcts are clinically silent, but a transient ischemic attack may occur in around 20% of patients

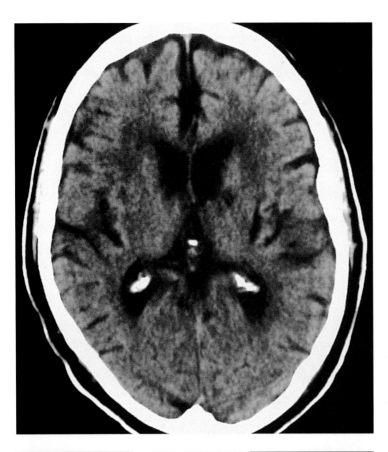

Figure 70 CT showing bilateral lacunar strokes in a 70-year-old patient with treatment-resistant hypertension and renal impairment due to hypertensive nephrosclerosis. The presenting features were a shuffling gait and pseudobulbar palsy

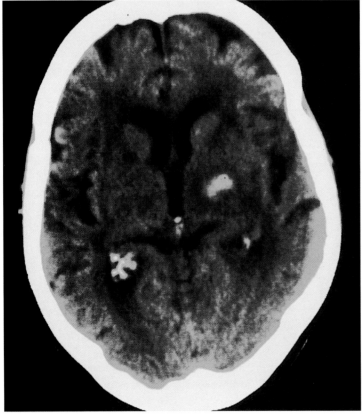

Figure 71 CT showing a small deep-lying hemorrhage which may present identically to lacunar infarction. In this case, the clinical presentation suggested a sensori-motor lacunar stroke. Both entities result from the occlusion and rupture, respectively, of perforating end arteries and are frequently due to hypertension

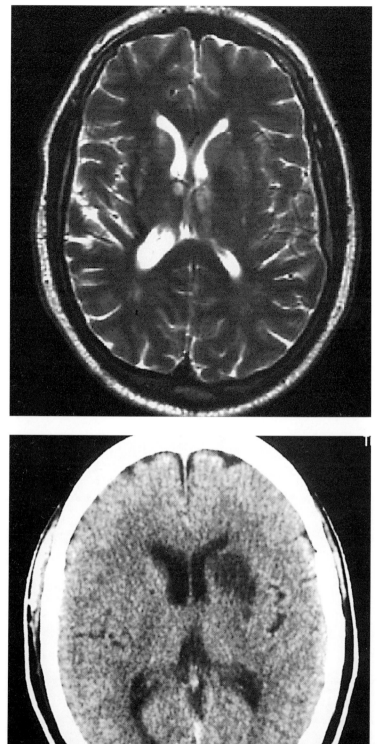

Figure 72 T$_2$-weighted MRI of a 60-year-old taxi driver, who had poorly controlled hypertension and previous right hemiparesis due to pure motor stroke, shows lacunar infarcts affecting the anterior poles of the thalamus, especially on the right. The patient presented with sudden-onset anterograde amnesia

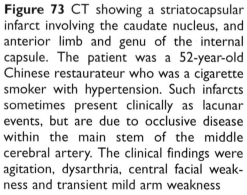

Figure 73 CT showing a striatocapsular infarct involving the caudate nucleus, and anterior limb and genu of the internal capsule. The patient was a 52-year-old Chinese restaurateur who was a cigarette smoker with hypertension. Such infarcts sometimes present clinically as lacunar events, but are due to occlusive disease within the main stem of the middle cerebral artery. The clinical findings were agitation, dysarthria, central facial weakness and transient mild arm weakness

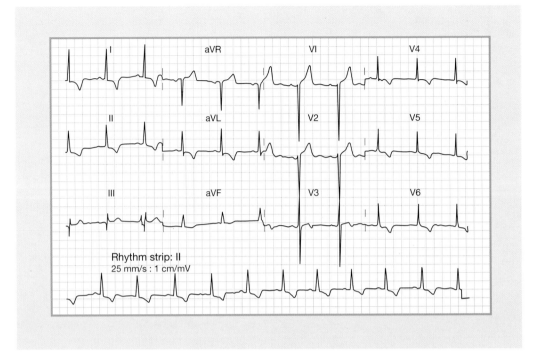

Figure 74 ECG in severe hypertension showing left ventricular hypertrophy by limb and chest lead-voltage criteria. Repolarization changes in the lateral leads or ST depression are often described as a 'strain' pattern: the S wave in V1 plus R wave in V5 >35 mm; the R wave in I plus S wave in III >25 mm; the R wave in aVL >11 mm

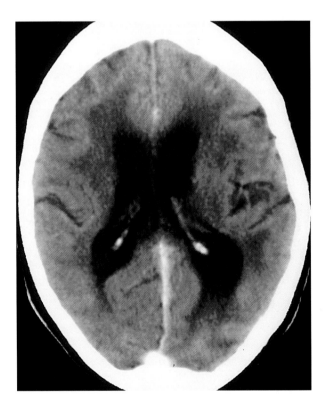

Figure 75 CT showing diffuse white-matter ischemia, which causes periventricular low attenuation. However, MRI is a more sensitive technique for visualizing these abnormalities. Age is the main predictor of this CT appearance

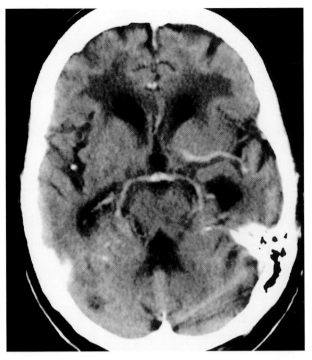

Figure 76 CT (same patient as in Figure 75) showing reduced attenuation around the anterior horns of the lateral ventricles

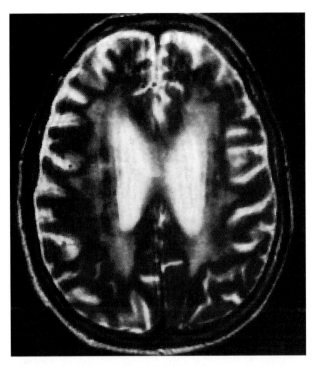

Figure 77 T$_2$-weighted MRI showing extensive periventricular white-matter ischemia in a 79-year-old patient who presented with a shuffling gait, abulia, bilateral pyramidal signs, primitive reflexes and mild memory loss. The appearances here are consistent with Binswanger's disease or microvascular ischemic leukoencephalopathy

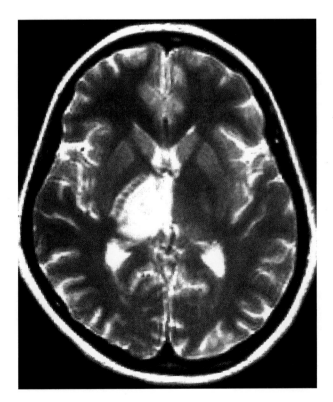

Figure 78 T$_2$-weighted MRI showing venous infarction, which often occurs in unusual situations. In this case, a 35-year-old woman presented, 3 days post-partum, with mild left brachiofacial weakness, sensory loss and headache. The infarct is large, deep and central on the right thalamus. MRI angiography showed occlusion of the straight venous sinus

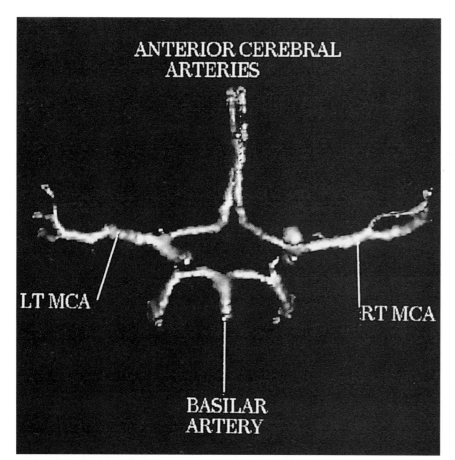

Figure 79 Three-dimensional surface reconstruction of a spiral CT shows a normal circle of Willis

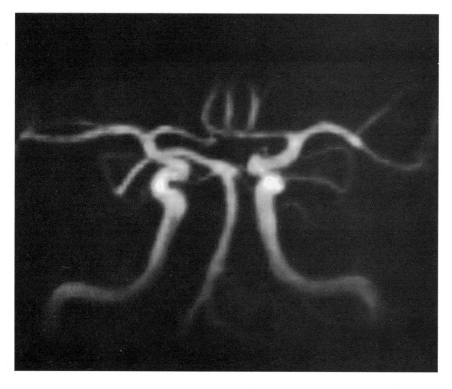

Figure 80 MRI angiography does not use contrast and is able to produce surprisingly good views of the circle of Willis, as seen in this normal examination. The definition, however, is not as good as with contrast arteriography

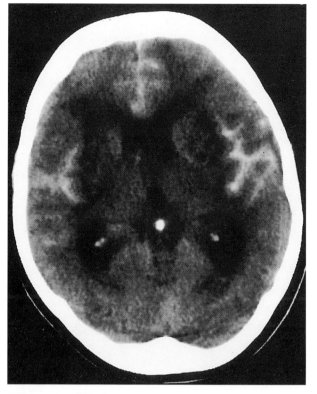

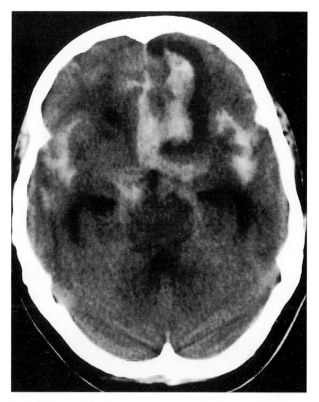

Figure 81 CT showing blood in the subarachnoid space in a 68-year-old patient who presented with sudden-onset severe headache and vomiting, followed by agitation and amnesia. Negative findings on CT do not exclude subarachnoid hemorrhage

Figure 82 CT (same patient as in Figure 81) at a lower cut shows hematoma that extends forwards from the midline to the ventromedial frontal lobe. These appearances are characteristic of rupture of an aneurysm of the anterior communicating artery

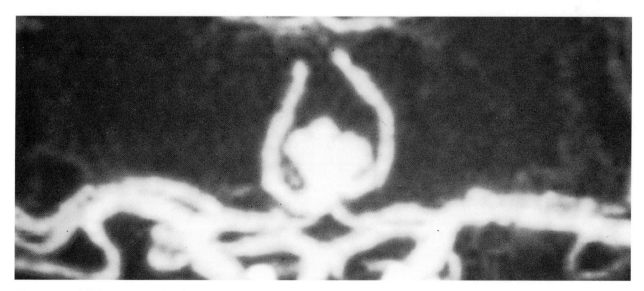

Figure 83 MRI angiography (same patient as in Figure 81) showing a large 'berry' aneurysm of the anterior communicating artery. The circle of Willis is viewed from behind

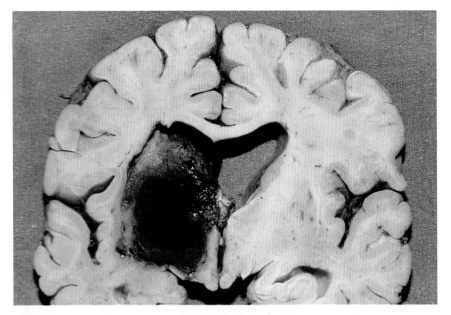

Figure 84 Coronal section through the cerebral cortex shows recent cerebral hemorrhage centered on the basal ganglia in a patient with hypertension. The bleeding probably originated from a ruptured microaneurysm

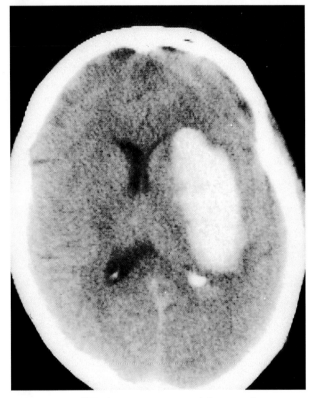

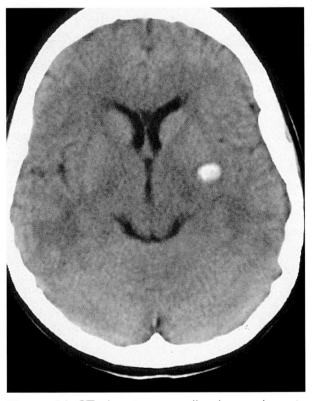

Figure 85 CT showing a typical hemorrhage into the putamen in a 43-year-old patient with undiagnosed hypertension presenting with abrupt onset of hemiplegia, hemisensory loss, hemianopia, global aphasia and forced deviation of gaze to the left. Bleeding originated in the lateral lenticulostriate territory often called the artery of cerebral hemorrhage

Figure 86 CT showing a smaller hemorrhage in a 59-year-old patient with hypertension who presented with contralateral pure motor hemiparesis. In such cases, CT is essential for the diagnosis

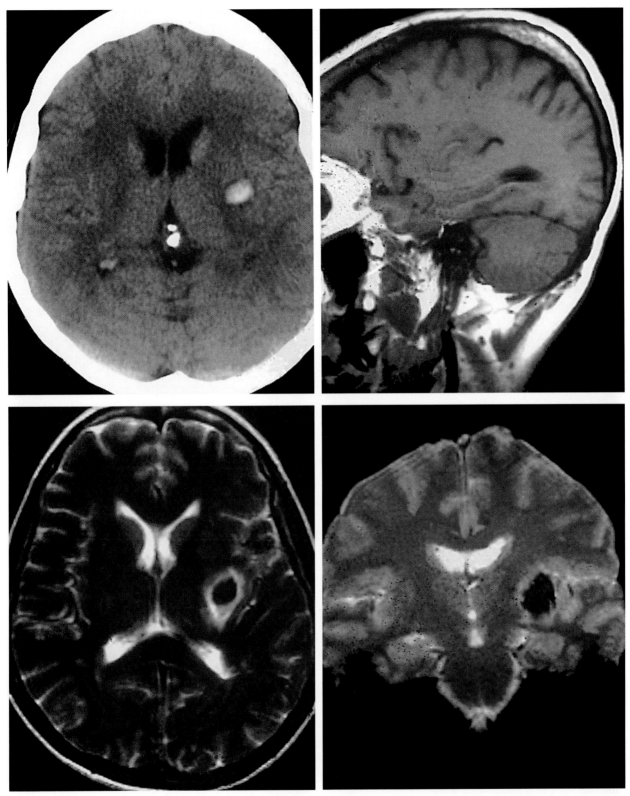

Figure 87 CT appearance of the hemorrhage (upper left) is compared with T_1-weighted (upper right) and T_2-weighted (lower) MRIs taken in three planes (same patient as in Figure 86) during the acute stage. Note the increased signal intensity caused by edema around the hematoma in the T_1-weighted image

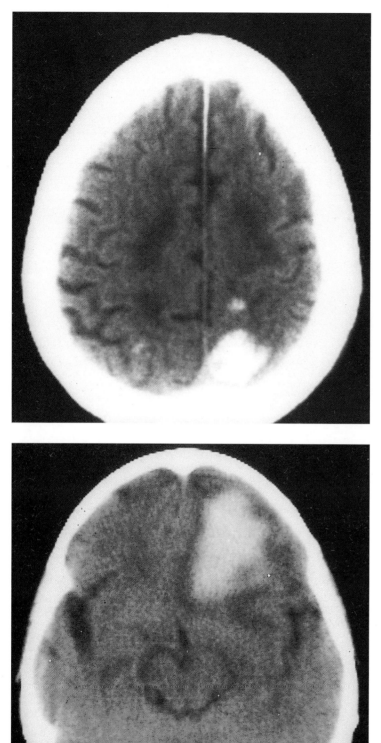

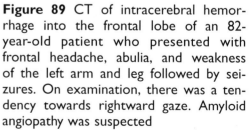

Figure 88 CT showing lobar intracerebral hemorrhage in the occipital cortex which presented as hemianopia, occipital headache and agitation in an 80-year-old patient. Bleeding at this age is often caused by amyloid angiopathy, which selectively affects small- and medium-sized arteries and veins of the cerebral cortex and pia mater

Figure 89 CT of intracerebral hemorrhage into the frontal lobe of an 82-year-old patient who presented with frontal headache, abulia, and weakness of the left arm and leg followed by seizures. On examination, there was a tendency towards rightward gaze. Amyloid angiopathy was suspected

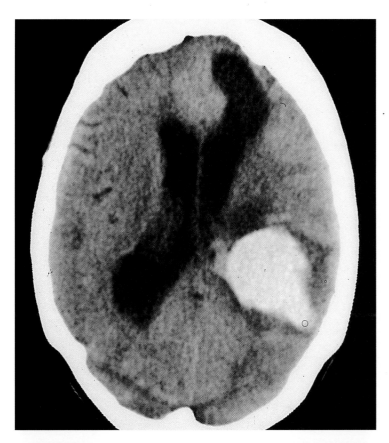

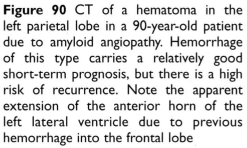

Figure 90 CT of a hematoma in the left parietal lobe in a 90-year-old patient due to amyloid angiopathy. Hemorrhage of this type carries a relatively good short-term prognosis, but there is a high risk of recurrence. Note the apparent extension of the anterior horn of the left lateral ventricle due to previous hemorrhage into the frontal lobe

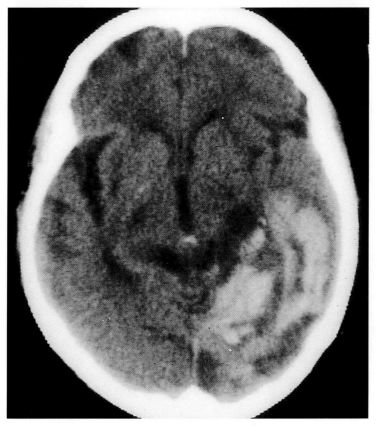

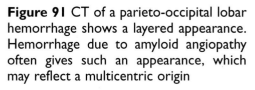

Figure 91 CT of a parieto-occipital lobar hemorrhage shows a layered appearance. Hemorrhage due to amyloid angiopathy often gives such an appearance, which may reflect a multicentric origin

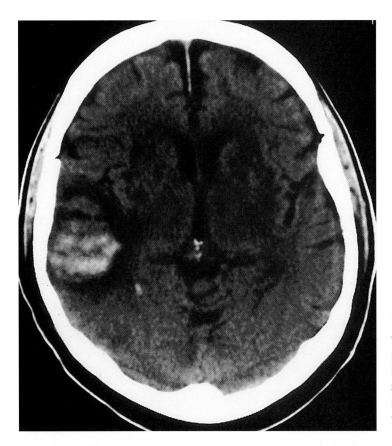

Figure 92 CT showing hemorrhage into the right parietal lobe of an 81-year-old patient treated with warfarin as prophylaxis for cerebral embolism due to atrial fibrillation. Lobar hemorrhage may be caused by fibrinolytic or anticoagulant treatment

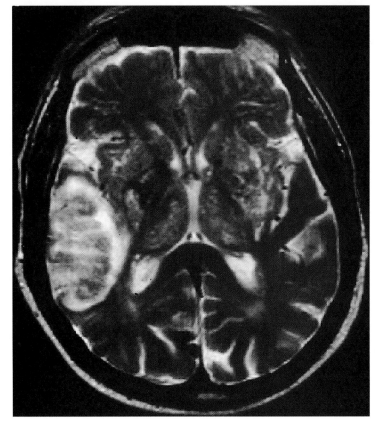

Figure 93 T_2-weighted MRI (same patient as in Figure 92) of the lobar hemorrhage in the subacute phase

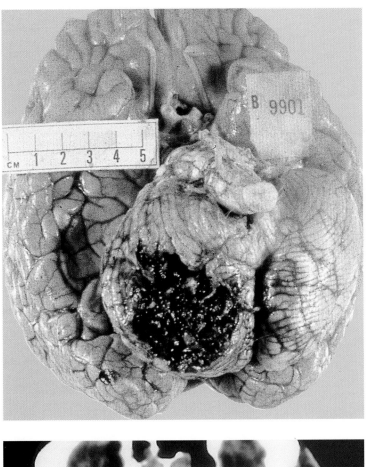

Figure 94 Brain viewed from the base showing hemorrhage into the right lobe of the cerebellum

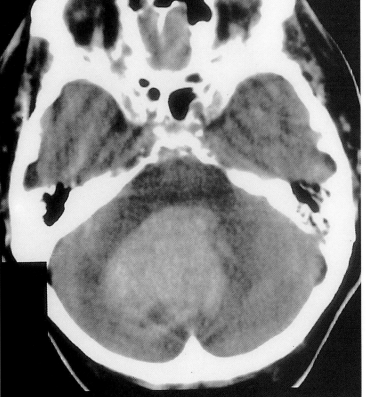

Figure 95 CT showing hemorrhage into the cerebellum, which may be caused by hypertension or amyloid angiopathy. The 62-year-old patient had poorly controlled hypertension and presented with collapse, inability to walk, occipital headache and vomiting. There was right-sided facial weakness of peripheral-type and gaze failure resulting from compression of the pons

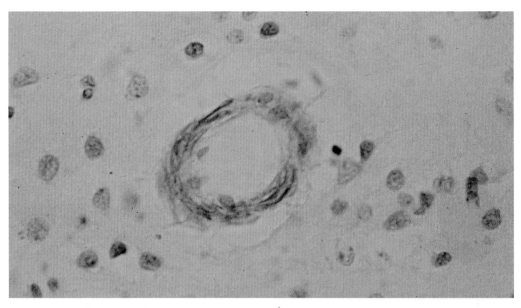

Figure 96 Histology of the cerebral cortex showing a vessel stained to reveal amyloid in the vessel walls (Congo red & hematoxylin)

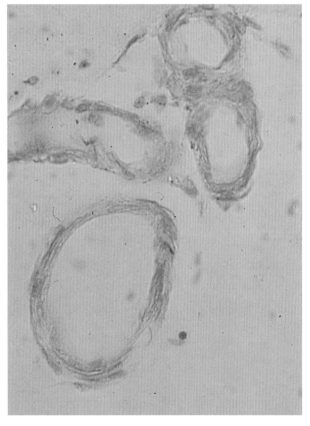

Figure 97 Histology of the leptomeninges showing vessels stained to reveal amyloid (Congo red & hematoxylin)

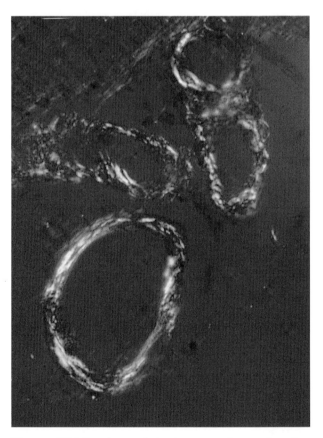

Figure 98 Histology of the leptomeninges showing vessels stained to reveal amyloid and viewed under polarized light to show the characteristic apple-green color (Congo red & hematoxylin)

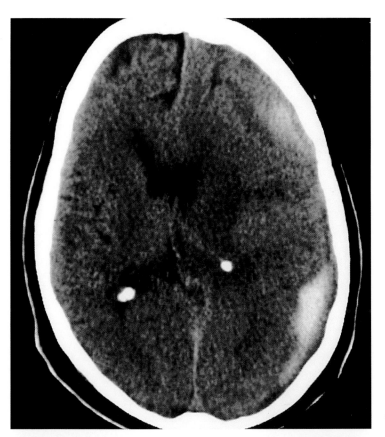

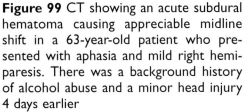

Figure 99 CT showing an acute subdural hematoma causing appreciable midline shift in a 63-year-old patient who presented with aphasia and mild right hemiparesis. There was a background history of alcohol abuse and a minor head injury 4 days earlier

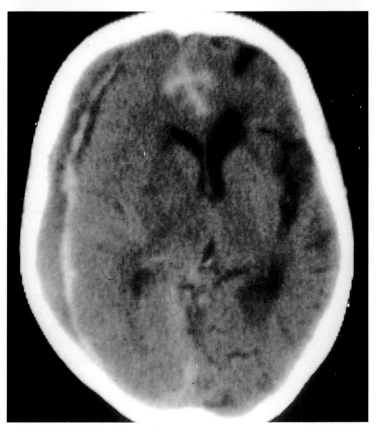

Figure 100 CT showing a less recent subdural hematoma which has become isodense with the brain tissue, although a hyperintense layer of more recent hemorrhage can still be seen adjacent to the cerebral cortex. Note the characteristic shape of the adjacent anterior horn of the lateral ventricle, which is often a clue to the presence of subdural blood on CT

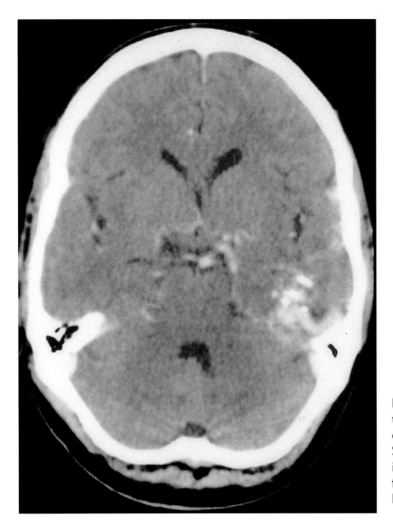

Figure 101 CT after intravenous injection of contrast shows a left parieto-occipital arteriovenous malformation. Such lesions often cause lobar hematoma in younger patients. In this case, the malformation appears to be supplied by the left posterior cerebral artery

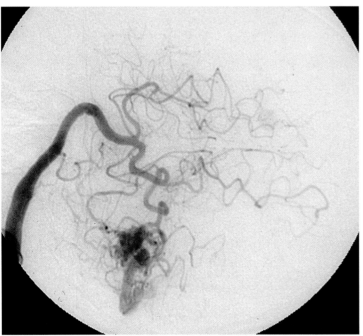

Figure 102 Contrast angiography (same patient as in Figure 101) of the vertebral artery confirms that the malformation is supplied by the left posterior cerebral artery. Lesions of this type also cause seizures

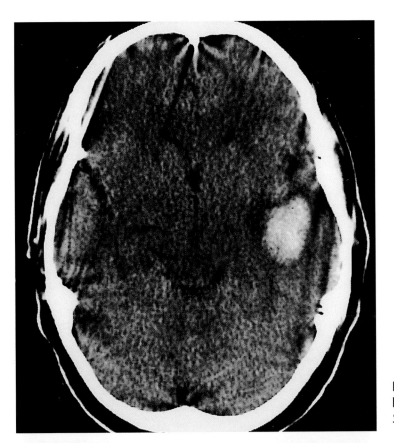

Figure 103 CT showing a left parietal hemorrhage in a 42-year-old patient with *Staphylococcus aureus* septicemia

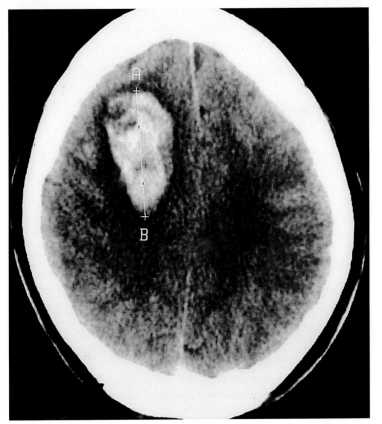

Figure 104 CT (same patient as in Figure 103) at a higher cut shows a separate large frontoparietal hemorrhage. Bleeding as a result of septic embolism tends to originate from the junction between gray and white matter

Index

References to illustrations are shown in **bold**.